CONTENTS

A REVIEW OF COMMUNITY HEALTH CENTERS: ISSUES AND OPPORTUNITIES

HEARING

BEFORE THE

SUBCOMMITTEE ON
OVERSIGHT AND INVESTIGATIONS

OF THE

COMMITTEE ON ENERGY AND COMMERCE
HOUSE OF REPRESENTATIVES

ONE HUNDRED NINTH CONGRESS

FIRST SESSION

MAY 25, 2005

Serial No. 109–31

Printed for the use of the Committee on Energy and Commerce

Available via the World Wide Web: http://www.access.gpo.gov/congress/house

U.S. GOVERNMENT PRINTING OFFICE

20–751PDF WASHINGTON : 2005

For sale by the Superintendent of Documents, U.S. Government Printing Office
Internet: bookstore.gpo.gov Phone: toll free (866) 512–1800; DC area (202) 512–1800
Fax: (202) 512–2250 Mail: Stop SSOP, Washington, DC 20402–0001

COMMITTEE ON ENERGY AND COMMERCE

JOE BARTON, Texas, *Chairman*

RALPH M. HALL, Texas
MICHAEL BILIRAKIS, Florida
Vice Chairman
FRED UPTON, Michigan
CLIFF STEARNS, Florida
PAUL E. GILLMOR, Ohio
NATHAN DEAL, Georgia
ED WHITFIELD, Kentucky
CHARLIE NORWOOD, Georgia
BARBARA CUBIN, Wyoming
JOHN SHIMKUS, Illinois
HEATHER WILSON, New Mexico
JOHN B. SHADEGG, Arizona
CHARLES W. "CHIP" PICKERING, Mississippi, *Vice Chairman*
VITO FOSSELLA, New York
ROY BLUNT, Missouri
STEVE BUYER, Indiana
GEORGE RADANOVICH, California
CHARLES F. BASS, New Hampshire
JOSEPH R. PITTS, Pennsylvania
MARY BONO, California
GREG WALDEN, Oregon
LEE TERRY, Nebraska
MIKE FERGUSON, New Jersey
MIKE ROGERS, Michigan
C.L. "BUTCH" OTTER, Idaho
SUE MYRICK, North Carolina
JOHN SULLIVAN, Oklahoma
TIM MURPHY, Pennsylvania
MICHAEL C. BURGESS, Texas
MARSHA BLACKBURN, Tennessee

JOHN D. DINGELL, Michigan
Ranking Member
HENRY A. WAXMAN, California
EDWARD J. MARKEY, Massachusetts
RICK BOUCHER, Virginia
EDOLPHUS TOWNS, New York
FRANK PALLONE, Jr., New Jersey
SHERROD BROWN, Ohio
BART GORDON, Tennessee
BOBBY L. RUSH, Illinois
ANNA G. ESHOO, California
BART STUPAK, Michigan
ELIOT L. ENGEL, New York
ALBERT R. WYNN, Maryland
GENE GREEN, Texas
TED STRICKLAND, Ohio
DIANA DEGETTE, Colorado
LOIS CAPPS, California
MIKE DOYLE, Pennsylvania
TOM ALLEN, Maine
JIM DAVIS, Florida
JAN SCHAKOWSKY, Illinois
HILDA L. SOLIS, California
CHARLES A. GONZALEZ, Texas
JAY INSLEE, Washington
TAMMY BALDWIN, Wisconsin
MIKE ROSS, Arkansas

BUD ALBRIGHT, *Staff Director*
DAVID CAVICKE, *Deputy Staff Director and General Counsel*
REID P.F. STUNTZ, *Minority Staff Director and Chief Counsel*

SUBCOMMITTEE ON OVERSIGHT AND INVESTIGATIONS

ED WHITFIELD, Kentucky, *Chairman*

CLIFF STEARNS, Florida
CHARLES W. "CHIP" PICKERING, Mississippi
CHARLES F. BASS, New Hampshire
GREG WALDEN, Oregon
MIKE FERGUSON, New Jersey
MICHAEL C. BURGESS, Texas
MARSHA BLACKBURN, Tennessee
JOE BARTON, Texas, (Ex Officio)

BART STUPAK, Michigan
Ranking Member
DIANA DEGETTE, Colorado
JAN SCHAKOWSKY, Illinois
JAY INSLEE, Washington
TAMMY BALDWIN, Wisconsin
HENRY A. WAXMAN, California
JOHN D. DINGELL, Michigan, (Ex Officio)

A REVIEW OF COMMUNITY HEALTH CENTERS: ISSUES AND OPPORTUNITIES

WEDNESDAY, MAY 25, 2005

HOUSE OF REPRESENTATIVES,
COMMITTEE ON ENERGY AND COMMERCE,
SUBCOMMITTEE ON OVERSIGHT AND INVESTIGATIONS,
Washington, DC.

The subcommittee met, pursuant to notice, at 2:03 p.m., in room 2322 of the Rayburn House Office Building, Hon. Ed Whitfield (chairman) presiding.

Members present: Representatives Whitfield, Stearns, Bass, Walden, Ferguson, Burgess, Blackburn, Barton (ex officio), Stupak, Inslee, Baldwin, and Waxman.

Also present: Representative Green.

Staff present: Anthony Cooke, majority counsel; Mark Paoletta, chief counsel; Chad Grant, legislative clerk; Jeanne Haggerty, majority counsel; Edith Hollman, minority counsel; and Voncille Hines, staff assistant.

Mr. WHITFIELD. At this time, I would like to call this hearing to order.

As you know, this is the Energy and Commerce Committee's Subcommittee on Oversight and Investigations, and today's hearing is entitled: "A Review of Community Health Centers." And I certainly want to thank all of those who will be participating today as witnesses.

And at this point, I will recognize myself for an opening statement.

We convene this afternoon to review community health centers. I look forward to today's hearing with particular interest, because I hope to bring, and I think this Subcommittee hopes to bring, national attention to the opportunities of this program for improving the lives and health of many Americans while at the same time bringing focus to the important role primary preventive health care can play in controlling health care costs.

To meet the promises we have made through the Medicaid and Medicare programs to provide health care we must always seek ways to use the taxpayers' money wisely and promoting preventing medicine for our most needy citizens is just one such opportunity.

I might also say that the President has recognized the promise of community health centers by placing them at the center of an initiative to expand the access and services of these important safety net institutions. Since 2002, this new funding to the community health center program has added the capacity to serve an additional 3 million Americans.

As the committee with principal authority over community health centers, we should look forward to learning directly from the health centers with us here today and to find out how this new money is going to work.

I might also say that when we decided to have this hearing, a lot of people were quite concerned, because they said, “Oh, my gosh. Why do they want to have a hearing about community health centers? Is it because their Congressional District does not have enough? Is it because they have got to find money to save in Medicaid? What is the reason?” And since I was one of those that thought up the idea of having it, and I know that Ranking Minority Member Stupak has had a real interest in this, and I know we have a witness from Michigan here today who is running a successful community health center, but my only interest was that, one, I don’t think that enough attention of the Congress has been focused on these health centers. And two, I think that they are providing an invaluable service in providing access to, particularly a lot of people who are uninsured, and I might add, uninsured people who do have jobs but whose employer is not paying their health care for them, and yet these people are paying the taxes so that people on Medicaid get their health coverage, people on Medicare get their health coverage, and they are paying their taxes, but yet they can’t afford to buy their own health coverage for their own families.

And so we wanted to focus on these community health centers. What are the opportunities out there for expansion? Are there some new initiatives that we may think of, new models that we could look at? You know, there are some unique things about these health centers. They do have some limited liability prospects under the Tort Claims Act. They get a discount on prescription drugs. So there are a lot of great attributes to these community health centers. And the real reason that we are having this hearing is simply to get a better understanding of how it works. Is there a well thought through policy on the relationship between the community health centers and Medicaid, between the community health centers and Medicare? Are there other avenues that we may need to go?

So I just wanted to mention that as a clarification. I certainly do not view this as a hearing of a way to save $10 billion next year for Medicaid. So I just want to set that in the record, set that straight. And I do look forward to the testimony, and what we might learn, and, hopefully, can come up with some conclusions that will help improve health care for everyone in America.

[The prepared statement of Hon. Ed Whitfield follows:]

PREPARED STATEMENT OF HON. ED WHITFIELD, CHAIRMAN, SUBCOMMITTEE ON OVERSIGHT AND INVESTIGATIONS

We convene this afternoon to review community health centers. I look forward to today’s hearing with particular interest because I hope to bring national attention to the opportunities of this program for improving the lives and health of many Americans while, at the same time, bringing focus to the important role primary, preventative health care can play in controlling health care costs. To meet the promises we have made through the Medicaid and Medicare programs to provide health care, we must always seek ways to use the taxpayers’ money wisely—and promoting preventative medicine for our most needy citizens is just one such opportunity.

Today there are over 900 community health centers providing a spectrum of primary health care services through 3600 urban and rural sites located in every state and territory. According to the Bureau of Primary Healthcare, community health centers in 2003 treated over 12 million people in medically underserved areas, including 4.8 million uninsured. Indeed, 90% of CHC patients live under 200% of the federal poverty line. In 2003, these community health centers delivered mammograms to over 200,000 women, gave check-ups and other health services to 1.6 million children and administered over 2.2 million immunizations. The primary healthcare services given by these community centers also included pre-natal care, mental health services, blood pressure and cholesterol checks and care of chronic diseases such as diabetes. I have a community health center in my District and know the vital role it plays in providing care to my constituents.

Community health centers play a critical role in our nation's healthcare safety net. The purpose of our oversight hearing today is to evaluate the effectiveness of the program in reaching the medically underserved and to listen to ideas that could build upon the program's areas of success. One such potential area of success, which is of particular interest in this time of tightening budgets, is the role of community health centers in giving the regular, preventative care that both enhances their patients' daily health but also keeps them out of hospitals and emergency rooms where the cost of providing care is more expensive. Healthy people naturally utilize fewer health care services thereby decreasing the burdens on our health care system and the Medicaid and Medicare programs. As one example, a study in 1980 found that a set of Medicaid patients, who used community health centers, had a 30% to 65% lower hospitalization rate and used 12% to 48% less total Medicaid funds than a similar group of Medicaid patients who did not use such health centers.

The President has also recognized the promise of community health centers by placing them at the center of an initiative to expand the access and services of these important safety net institutions. Since 2002, this new funding to the community health center program has added the capacity to serve an additional 3 million Americans. As the Committee with principal authority over community health centers, we should look forward to learning directly from the health centers with us here today how this new money is going to work.

Finally, I would note here that there is surprisingly little recent research on the issue of whether community health centers create savings to our public health programs such as Medicaid, through their provision of preventative care. As such, I recently asked the Government Accountability Office to study this important connection and I look forward to its report.

I welcome today's witnesses and appreciate their appearance here. I hope this hearing will leave us all with a more complete understanding of the community health center program and ways in which it might better serve the medically underserved of this nation while, at the same time, helping to control overall healthcare costs.

Mr. WHITFIELD. And with that, I yield back the balance of my time and recognize the gentleman from Michigan, Mr. Stupak.

Mr. STUPAK. Thank you, Mr. Chairman, and thank you for holding this hearing.

First, I want to welcome Kim Sibilsky, the Executive Director of the Michigan Primary Health Care Association, who has dedicated many, many years to making sure that Michigan has one of the best community health care systems in the country. I look forward to hearing her testimony today.

Community health centers are one of the few success stories in the health care field. They provide quality primary care at a fraction of the cost to the uninsured, but also provide care to the insured. Not only are community health centers the epitome of doing more with less by being incredibly resourceful in using the funding they receive, but also community health centers lower the costs of health care overall by keeping people out of the hospital emergency rooms where the cost of care is much greater. As a result, the community health care program continues to enjoy strong, bipartisan support.

Under both the Clinton and Bush Administrations, Congress has expanded the budget and the geographic coverage of these centers. In the most recent dismal health care disparities report of 2004, which I have placed in the exhibit book, the Department of Health and Human Services reports ever decreasing quality of care and less access for most disadvantaged and poor groups except those who receive care in community health centers.

But community health centers face serious challenges. The linchpin that keeps these centers financially afloat is the Medicaid reimbursement. About one-third of their income comes from Medicaid. Along with the base Federal grant and SCHIP, Medicaid is what allows these centers to care for the uninsured, those who have limited health care insurance, and those with no place else to go. Yet Medicaid is under attack. The Energy and Commerce Committee has been ordered to cut Medicaid by $15 billion to $20 billion over 5 years. This cut is equivalent to completely eliminating Federal funding for Medicaid coverage between 1.8 and 2.5 low-income parents for each of the next 5 years. States simply can not afford these cuts. Michigan's high unemployment rate makes Ms. Sibilsky's job and that of rural health centers and federally qualified health centers more difficult. This is especially true with Medicaid cuts expected to be between $15 billion to $20 billion.

The fact is that States are already struggling, making cuts, and impacting the community health centers. When States decide to reduce their Medicaid roles or cut coverage services, the community's health centers can't throw out these people or stop providing care. The patients still need health care, and the centers are legally obligated to provide it. When States cut Medicaid, the community health centers are hit with a double whammy: community health centers lose Medicaid payments for their current patients and community health centers get new patients who are being turned away from or can't afford their private providers.

Attached to my statement is an overview of how Michigan community health centers are being hit. Michigan, for example, stopped paying for dental care for adult Medicaid patients. But that service is more utilized than any other by patients in the State's community health care centers. They have to keep providing it. The poor oral health has serious long-term effects on people's health, morbidity, and employability. But who will pay for it?

Who also will pay for the health care of those whose employers can no longer afford it? Many employers are struggling to compete in the global economy and can no longer offer affordable health insurance to their employees. When employers cut insurance coverage, the burden falls to Medicaid and community health centers. Twenty-seven percent of the adults on Medicaid in Michigan have a job. Ms. Sibilsky says it better than I could: "When you restrict enrollment in public programs, the cost to providing care does not disappear and the savings are not absolute. People will eventually receive the care they need. It may not be in the best and most cost-effective location at a time when progression of illness can be headed off and the most expensive care prevented, but in the end, anyone can walk into a community hospital and receive some level of care." Michigan centers are already confronting higher co-payments, longer waiting periods for new patients, reduction in services, and losses in the hundreds of thousands of dollars for ineligible oral health care. Community health centers face still more challenges. Who is going to provide the money for capital expenditures, something the Federal Government doesn't pay for? A number of these centers are becoming very adept at private fundraising, but more and more often they are competing with other worthy causes, which are losing their funding because of shortsighted political decisions made here in Washington. The centers need computers, equipment, expanded facilities, and staff.

The President has a commendable goal of creating many new health centers, but we can't improve health care if the tradeoff is letting the existing centers stay barely alive. In addition, the President's budget slashes funding from $300 million this year to $11 million next year for the Health Professions Program, which specifically provides Federal funding to bring physicians and other health care providers to under-served populations, the exact same populations served by community health centers.

It is distressing, Mr. Chairman, to see a program that is so successful, so efficient, so economical, and so praised face problems of this size and complexity. I hope this hearing today will provide more than a feel-good experience for the members and we begin to discuss how arbitrary budget cuts in Washington directly affect our ability to provide quality health care and coverage to those most in need.

Mr. Chairman, I yield back the balance of my time.

Mr. WHITFIELD. Thank you, Mr. Stupak.

At this time, I will recognize the gentleman from Oregon, Mr. Walden, for his opening statement.

Mr. WALDEN. Well, thank you very much, Mr. Chairman. I appreciate your holding this hearing. I have been a big advocate of the centers. I spent 5 years on a community hospital board, chaired and worked on committees in the Oregon legislature and enacted the Oregon Health Plan in an effort to better serve and better utilize Medicaid funding to try and do preventive work as well.

I hadn't planned to get into the argument over Medicaid funding, but just for the record, I believe the target that we have to achieve on all areas within our jurisdiction in this committee is something to the order of $10 billion and not $15 billion. And we do have other ways we can generate revenues, too, from things like spectrum auction.

I would also point out that we did support, as I recall on the floor and in the budget resolution that has been passed, the Medicaid Commission is due to report on how we can achieve greater efficiencies in Medicaid. And as an employer, I certainly sympathize with the cost of health care. My own insurance policies in my company, premiums went up close to 20 percent this year. So there are a lot of conflicting pressures on health care delivery, and it is our opportunity and challenge to figure out how best to take care of people who need health care in the most efficient and affordable way possible. And it is not through the emergency room door. It is through clinics like this.

And I want to brag a bit in terms of what has happened in my home State of Oregon, where we have 23 community health centers which support over 125 sites in urban, rural, and frontier areas.

Now I want to talk about a frontier area. My District is the second biggest in the Nation other than the five single-member States. And let us cut to the chase and go right on out to Wheeler County where there are 1,713 square miles. That is about the same as the population in the county. Okay. That is the size an area as big as the State of Rhode Island. And located there is the Asher Clinic, the sole life-saving source for health care. The two surrounding counties of Wheeler County, Sherman and Gilliam, none of these three counties has a hospital. They have clinics. They have physician assistants. One, I guess, now has a doctor but for many years didn't. This clinic out in Wheeler County faced some difficulty and initial rejection to be able to get qualified as a Federal health center and was facing a shortfall of $80,000 a year. That is a huge sum in a community like that, a county of 1,700 people or thereabouts. So they contacted me and my staff in May 2003, and we helped them work through some of the paperwork and all, and I really want to commend Elizabeth Duke and her folks for their work on this effort as well, because they were, in 2004, able to receive a health center grant for $229,500, and you would have thought they won the $100 million lottery. And I went out to Wheeler County not long after that to help them celebrate a bit. And you know, we really are talking about life saving, a source of health care. Because you can drive, in parts of my District, 100 miles in any direction before you hit the first stop light. And if you have a crisis in health care, if clinics like this don't exist, you are out of luck unless you wait for a helicopter to come pick you up and transport you somewhere, which is the alternative, or you race in a car somewhere to try and find health care.

And so I am a firm believer in these federally qualified clinics. I believe they can be, and are, a very productive way to help people who don't have health insurance get care before it is an emergency and improve their own qualities of life.

So Mr. Chairman, I appreciate your oversight on this. We are spending a lot of money in this area. It is our obligation to look at what is working and what is not, as we do in this subcommittee and as you do very aggressively as our chairman. And I think it is good to point out once in a while where things are working and use, as an example, these clinics, and if there are problems, let us figure out where things work better and apply those standards elsewhere. But we have got big challenges in this Congress when it comes to the delivery of health care services. And if you add up the promises that have been made from Social Security, Medicare, and Medicaid, we bankrupt the next generation if we don't get it right now.

And so hopefully, as we look at issues involving, for example, the work this subcommittee has done on AWP versus ASP on how we pay for drugs versus what it costs to actually get them. There are some false economies there and actually some perverse incentives to drive up costs of pharmaceuticals to Medicaid and robs money, I believe, from actually being able to expand and deliver service. It could be as much as $15 billion over 10 years. These are issues that we have looked at in this committee and need to look at closely as we try to reform Medicaid to be able to deliver the most service most efficiently to the most number of people.

And so I welcome this hearing, and I appreciate your and our staff's work in this area.

And I yield back the remaining 3½ seconds.

Mr. WHITFIELD. Thank you, Mr. Walden, for being so generous with your time.

And Mr. Waxman, you are recognized for your opening statement.

Mr. WAXMAN. Thank you very much, Mr. Chairman.

Well, it is clear from what I have heard so far that there is strong, bipartisan support for the community health centers. It is one of the real successes of our Federal health policy.

But I want to make one point that Mr. Stupak indicated. We will be doing a real disservice to the community health centers if we make some of the cuts in Medicaid that are being proposed. It may not be the $15 billion or $20 billion, although we still don't know if somebody might just come up with something more than $10 billion, but $10 billion is not a small amount of money. It is the Medicaid program that is the lifeblood of these centers. If we had not established the federally Qualified Health Centers Program in Medicaid in 1989 guaranteeing community health centers that they would be covered providers in the Medicaid program and reimbursed at a fair level that recognized their costs, many centers just would not be viable. And it is hard to praise those centers when they are not around anymore. It is a crucial source of payment, and they are not going to be around anymore if we make some of these cuts in Medicaid.

If we cut the Medicaid program and we take away the guarantee of coverage for eligible people, we will be damaging the community health center program just as directly as if we slashed its funding. If we accede to State calls for flexibility and take away the payment and coverage guarantees we have given to FQHCs, then it is the viability of the community health centers that will be directly threatened.

It is easy to voice support for these centers but miss the crucial link to a robust Medicaid program. Certainly the administration, in my view, has been hypocritical in touting their support for community health centers while they work for constant changes in Medicaid, which would damage these institutions beyond repair.

In addition to Medicaid, community health centers see the uninsured. Well, we will have many more uninsured if there is not a Medicaid eligibility for them to get that coverage. We will have more uninsured, less payment, and the community health centers, and other providers, will not be able to absorb those costs.

I thank you, Mr. Chairman, for holding this hearing. Let us keep all of these things in mind, because there are a lot of times we don't want the unforeseen consequences to occur when we adopt legislation, but let us take the time in this Oversight Committee to foresee what would happen if we make short-term cuts in Medicaid to deal with the budget and then have very foreseen consequences that could be so harmful to a program that has been working well.

Mr. WHITFIELD. Mr. Ferguson, do you have an opening statement? And while you are preparing, I would like to recognize and welcome Mr. Green of Texas, who is a member of the Energy and

Commerce Committee. He does not happen to be a member of this subcommittee, but we know of his intense interest in community health centers and welcome him here today. It is the policy of the subcommittee that if you are not a member of the subcommittee, you can not make an opening statement, but you can certainly ask questions and make comments during that period. And I know you are excited about the number of health centers in Texas, and I was going to be really astute and give you the number, but now I can't seem to find it, but I think there are something like 35 grantees, or so, in Texas.

But at this time, I recognize Mr. Ferguson for his 5-minute opening statement.

Mr. FERGUSON. Thank you, Mr. Chairman.

I am sorry I was walking in a couple of minutes late.

I want to thank you for holding this hearing about an initiative that has received great support from the President and the administration and is currently providing care to millions of poor and under-served Americans in our country today. In a short time, community health centers have emerged as viable sources of health care for the poor of our Nation. In fact, 90 percent of people that have used community health centers are people under 200 percent of the Federal poverty level. Community health centers in 2003 treated over 12 million people in medically under-served areas, including 4.8 million uninsured patients. That same year, 1.6 million children received check-ups or other health services from CHCs and they administered over 2.2 million immunizations. Pre-natal care, mental health services, blood pressure, mammograms, and cholesterol checks and care of chronic diseases, such as diabetes, all take place at community health centers every day.

All of these statistics are impressive, but we can do more. I am thankful that we are going to have this opportunity today to delve into what we can do to help make community health centers serve the community better. For instance, is it possible to open up the grant process to faith-based groups to help provide these health services to the poor and under-served? Today, for instance, there are over 500 Catholic-sponsored health clinics for the poor, serving the exact same patient population as community health centers, but they are not eligible for Federal funding.

I thank the chairman for holding this important hearing. I look forward to hearing from our expert panel. And I welcome their suggestions.

Thank you, Mr. Chairman. I yield back.

Mr. WHITFIELD. Thank you, Mr. Ferguson.

At this time, I recognize Ms. Baldwin for her opening statement.

Ms. BALDWIN. Thank you, Mr. Chairman.

I want to commend you for holding today's hearing on community health centers.

Like my colleagues, I, too, am a strong supporter of community health centers and their mission. I represent a District with two federally qualified health centers, and I like to visit them frequently. I am constantly impressed with the excellent job that they do with extremely limited resources. I think each of us knows the large role that community health centers play in responding to the health needs of our uninsured, our under-insured, and low-income constituents and other targeted communities within our constituency.

But the community health centers are also the first to talk with me when I visit about the unmet needs that exist in our community that they are simply not able to meet, the people that they must turn away on a daily, weekly, and monthly basis. As just one example, because of the fact that no dentist in the largest county in the District that I represent has accepted new Medicaid patients in over 2 years, the Madison Community Health Center has tried very hard to fill some of that role. They have just expanded and moved into a new building with dental suites. They can currently serve over 12,000 individuals per year who need dental care, but it is estimated that 63,000 more people in that one county need dental care but don't receive it.

There are two closing points that I want to make. Even acknowledging what a huge fan I am of community health centers and the incredible job that they do in our community, I just want to say that they are clearly a response to the crisis of uninsurance in our country, but in my view, not the solution. And I remain committed to the belief that this Congress ought to declare health care to be a right and not a privilege, that we ought to ultimately tackle the challenge of universal health care.

Also, I want to underscore what several other colleagues have said in their opening statements about my strong concerns on how community health centers will be impacted by the impending cuts anticipated in the Medicaid program. Obviously, we all agree that community health centers' role and mission are vital, and at a time when the situation is so dire, we need them to have the capacity to respond to as many in need as possible.

With that, Mr. Chairman, I yield back my remaining time.

Mr. WHITFIELD. Thank you, Ms. Baldwin.

At this time, I will recognize the gentleman from Texas, Dr. Burgess, for his opening statement.

Mr. BURGESS. Thank you, Mr. Chairman.

The District that I represent actually has just crossed the finish line with its first community health center. My District is truly a cross-section of the country. Within its boundaries, you will find a mix of rich, poor, middle income, rural, suburban, urban, black, Anglo, and Hispanic citizens. You will also see sharp differences in the health needs of different communities and how they are impacted by the very health disparities.

For instance, in one part of my District, you will see some of the highest infant mortality rates anywhere in the country, and indeed, higher than some areas in parts of the world that we feel are less developed. In other parts of my District, the population is healthier but without ready access to health insurance. A new community health center in Denton, Texas is beginning to make a difference by giving community residents access to a physician at free or reduced cost. This will not only improve their short-term health, but will help with the creation of a medical home.

I am also actively seeking out stakeholders in the city of Fort Worth to look at standing up a clinic in Southeast Fort Worth to meet the needs of this community. This area of Fort Worth, having yet to really catch the wave of economic development that has benefited other areas of the city, is crying out for the type of assistance that a community health center can provide.

As we proceed from this hearing, I hope to be able to tap some of the expertise here in the room and assist my constituents that look to establish a community health center back home.

Thank you, Mr. Chairman, for calling this hearing, and I will yield back.

Mr. WHITFIELD. I thank you, Dr. Burgess.

At this time, I recognize the gentleman from New Hampshire for his opening statement.

Mr. BASS. Thank you, Mr. Chairman.

This is an interesting hearing. Community health care centers are a very important part of almost every Congressional District and every State in the country. I have the benefit of having at least three or four in my District. I believe there are seven altogether in the State of New Hampshire. And what they do, as may have been mentioned before, is provide a bridge for adequate health care between those who qualify for Medicaid and those that buy a health insurance policy. I note that the budget for community health care centers has gone up almost double in the last 4 or 5 years because we recognize, as does the administration, this is an important part of the whole health care picture in this country.

It is a good hearing, a good time for a hearing. I will be interested to know whether there are any issues involved with whether the competitive bidding process or application process for grants ends up resulting in having lots of community health care centers in some parts of the country or in some States and not in others where they may be needed.

So Mr. Chairman, I appreciate your calling this hearing, and I look forward to hearing from the witnesses.

Mr. WHITFIELD. Thank you, Mr. Bass.

And I am going to ask unanimous consent that we also enter into the record about nine documents that specifically relate to the health centers. The staffs on both sides of the aisle have reviewed this, and I think it will be helpful to complete the record with that.

So without objection, these documents, a total of nine of them, will be entered into the record.

[The information referred to appears at the end of the hearing.]

Mr. WHITFIELD. We are going to pause for just 1 minute. I have been told that the Chairman of the Full Committee is on his way, and I know that he did want to make an opening statement. So I am going to ask for your patience for a minute. We will see if he is going to be here.

Mr. GREEN. Mr. Chairman, while we are waiting for the opening statement, could I just ask unanimous consent to place a statement into the record?

Mr. WHITFIELD. Yes. That will be fine.

Thank you, Mr. Green.

While we are waiting on the Chairman, I would like, at this time, to call the first panel to the witness stand.

The first panel consists of Dr. Elizabeth Duke, who is the Administrator of Health Resources and Services Administration with the U.S. Department of Health and Human Services. Dr. Duke, we are delighted that you are here with us today, and we look forward to your testimony. In addition, Mr. Dennis Smith, who is the Director of the Center for Medicaid and State Operation, the Centers for Medicare and Medicaid Services at the U.S. Department of Health and Human Services.

So we do welcome you all here today.

And at this time, the Chairman of the Full Energy and Commerce Committee, Mr. Joe Barton of Texas, has just arrived. And I know he has a specific interest in community health centers. And at this time, we would recognize him for his opening statement.

Chairman BARTON. Well, first, Mr. Chairman, happy birthday to you.

If I had known a little bit sooner, we would have had a cake, but you are now old enough to vote, and we appreciate that.

Mr. WHITFIELD. I am 52 today.

Chairman BARTON. Today is your birthday, so happy birthday.

I need to give Congressman Ferguson, Mr. Embryo himself, credit for that. You know, we were all embryos once, and that is going to be on your tombstone.

But to get to the subject of today's hearing, Mr. Chairman, community health centers get little national attention. As the chairman of the committee with direct jurisdiction over the program, I personally want to learn more about how these centers work, what role they actually play in delivering health care, and what cost savings they might achieve. And I believe, Mr. Chairman, this hearing is one of the first hearings any committee of the Congress has held on community health centers in a long, long time, and I want to commend you for that.

The program itself is decades old. It was intended then and now to serve the poor. It was a small program, but now it is a large one. We operate over 3,600 urban and rural size in every State and Territory, and community health centers serve more than 12 million people.

I am interested in knowing more about the care offered by these centers and the impact that they have on both patients and the general health care system in America.

It has been reported that community health centers lower the cost of Medicaid. We are told that even as far back as 1980 there was a study that found a set of Medicaid patients who use community health centers use between 12 to 48 percent less total Medicaid funds than a similar group of Medicaid patients who did not use community health centers. That is back in 1980. Well, now we are in 2005. Is the same thing true today?

I am also interested in learning whether community health centers have been successful or can be successful in moving routine patient care out of emergency rooms to clinics where the quality is better and the care costs are dramatically lower.

The President has also included community health centers in his domestic health care agenda, and the President's initiative since 2001 has increased the number of community health centers by 334. As the primary authorizing committee, we must remain informed about how these additional centers have been allocated around the country.

I really want to thank you, Mr. Chairman, on your birthday, for holding this hearing. I look forward to the committee's review, and we look forward to moving forward, possibly in legislative areas, if this hearing shows that we need to.

With that, I yield back.

[The prepared statement of Hon. Joe Barton follows:]

PREPARED STATEMENT OF HON. JOE BARTON, CHAIRMAN, COMMITTEE ON ENERGY AND COMMERCE

The subject of today's hearing, community health centers, seems to get little national attention. But, over a number of years, these centers have been slowly building a track record that suggests promising developments in the difficult area of health care. Community health centers have seemed to be both helping patients live healthier lives while, at the same time, controlling overall costs. Like any member of Congress hearing something like this—I want to learn more. And as Chairman of the Committee with direct jurisdiction over this program—I want to find how to support the good work of these centers.

The community health center program is not new. Indeed it has its roots in efforts during the 1960's to promote health services within underserved communities. Bypassing the bureaucracies of state governments, federal money went directly to community based organizations delivering basic health services to some of the most needy among us.

Today, this effort continues in over 900 community health centers which operate 3600 urban and rural sites in every state and territory and serve over 12 million people. In 2003, these community health centers delivered mammograms to over 200,000 women, gave check-ups and other health services to 1.6 million children and administered over 2.2 million immunizations. Pre-natal care, mental health services, blood pressure and cholesterol checks—all to a patient population 90% of whom lived under 200% of poverty. I am interested in learning more about the care offered by these centers and looking at ways, such as through extended hours, to enhance access to these services.

While these centers have made important differences in the lives and health of their patients, there may also be good news about the role these centers play in the health of our vital Medicaid and Medicare programs. As one example, a study in 1980 found that a set of Medicaid patients, who used community health centers, had a 30% to 65% lower hospitalization rate and used 12% to 48% less total Medicaid funds than a similar group of Medicaid patients who did not use such health centers. In other words: an ounce of prevention may, indeed, be worth a pound of cure. Community health centers treat people preventatively in a doctor's office instead of finding them in the more expensive setting of an emergency room. This lowers costs to programs such as Medicaid without sacrificing the quality of the health care delivered to beneficiaries.

The President has made support and expansion of Community Health Centers a priority in his domestic health care agenda. For example, since 2001, the President's Initiative has increased the number of community health center sites by 334 locations. As the primary authorizing Committee, we must remain well informed of developments in this program and be ready to seize opportunities to leverage and apply more broadly the good ideas they have developed.

I thank the Chairman of the Subcommittee, Ed Whitfield, for holding this hearing today. I look forward to the Committee's review of community health centers and the chance to look at the issues and opportunities involved in this program.

Mr. WHITFIELD. And thank you, Mr. Chairman.

At this time, I recognize the gentlelady from Tennessee, Ms. Blackburn, for her opening statement.

Ms. BLACKBURN. Thank you, Mr. Chairman.

And I want to thank you, also, for holding this hearing.

And I want to thank the witnesses for taking the opportunity to come and talk with us about the community health center program. I know Mr. Smith is a little familiar with my District. He has been on the road with me in that District. And you know we have some fine community health centers there. And we thank you for your time today.

And as we look at this issue, I want us to carefully examine the effectiveness of the centers, because these centers provide direct health care services for some of America's population that is most in need of quality, low-cost health care. And having that access is important.

As the cost of health care has been dramatically rising over the past decade, this committee must ensure that these health centers are performing adequately and in the most cost-efficient manner before we dedicate new funding for the program. I look forward to the responses from these agencies on how the health centers are conducting risk management training and implementation of efforts for quality performance reviews that minimize the risk of malpractice claims and medical liability.

And again, I thank you very much for your time.

And Mr. Chairman, I thank you for the hearing.

Mr. WHITFIELD. And I have already introduced our witnesses on the first panel.

As you are aware, this is an investigative hearing, and it is the practice of this subcommittee that when we hold hearings, that the witnesses testify under oath. And I would ask the two of you, do you have any difficulty testifying under oath this afternoon?

Ms. DUKE. No.

Mr. SMITH. No.

Mr. WHITFIELD. I would also advise you that you do have the right to counsel if you want counsel, and I am assuming that neither one of you have legal counsel with you today. So in that case, if you would please rise and raise your right hand, I will swear you in.

[Witnesses sworn.]

Mr. WHITFIELD. Thank you.

I will proudly tell you, now you are officially sworn in. And Dr. Duke, we will begin with you, and you may give your 5-minute opening statement.

TESTIMONY OF ELIZABETH M. DUKE, ADMINISTRATOR, HEALTH RESOURCES AND SERVICES ADMINISTRATION, U.S. DEPARTMENT OF HEALTH AND HUMAN SERVICES; AND DENNIS SMITH, DIRECTOR, CENTER FOR MEDICAID AND STATE OPERATIONS, CENTERS FOR MEDICARE & MEDICAID SERVICES, U.S. DEPARTMENT OF HEALTH AND HUMAN SERVICES

Ms. DUKE. Thank you very much, sir.

I would like to submit the longer statement for the record and just give an abbreviated statement, if I may.

I want to thank you very much for having this hearing and for allowing us to be with you this afternoon.

You know that the health centers, in 2004, served an estimated 13.2 million people. That was about 3 million more than they served in 2001. And they did that service at 3,650 service delivery sites, which represents an increase of 600 new and expanded sites since 2001. In 2005, we plan to fund 153 new or expanded health center sites and to serve almost 14 million people.

The President's 2006 budget request includes an additional $277 million to complete the President's 5-year health center initiative by increasing the number of health center sites by 275 and significantly expanding 303 existing sites to increase the number of people served by 2.4 million above the 2005 level for a total of 16.3 million patients.

The President has also set a new goal to open a health center or a rural health clinic in every poor county that can support one. The budget includes a $26 million request to open new health center sites in 40 of the Nation's poorest counties and will support 25 planning grants as well. The goal of this initiative is to leverage the success of the current program to poor counties that can support a health center and provide access to primary and preventive health care services, particularly in poor counties that are medically under-served.

The distinguishing mission of the health center program is to empower communities to solve their own local access problems and to improve the health status of their under-served and vulnerable populations by building community-based primary care capacity and by offering case management, home visiting, outreach, and other enabling services.

The program also addresses significant challenges facing communities by targeting public housing, homeless, and migrant health center development as well. Health centers can provide access to high-quality, family oriented, comprehensive primary and preventive care regardless of ability to pay.

Health center grantees, as a result of their receiving a HRSA grant, under Section 330 of the Public Health Service Act, are eligible for enhanced benefits, including Medicaid and Medicare reimbursement, access to the Federal Tort Claims Act program for malpractice coverage and access to the program for discount drugs for patients under Section 340B of the PHS Act.

Under Section 330, a health center is required to provide primary health services, including those related to family medicine, internal medicine, pediatrics, obstetrics, or gynecology, that are furnished by physicians and, where appropriate, physicians assistants, nurse practitioners, and nurse midwives. Additionally, they are required to have basic health services, including diagnostic laboratory and radiological services and services in preventive health.

To receive Section 330 grant funds, a clinic must meet a number of statutory requirements. The health center must be located in a federally designated medically under-served area or serve a federally designated medically under-served population. It must also be a public or a private non-private health center, provide comprehensive primary health services, referrals, and other services needed to facilitate access to care, such as case management, translation, and transportation. It must have a governing board, the majority of whose members are patients of the health center, provide services to all in the area regardless of their ability to pay, and offer a sliding fee schedule that adjusts according to individual family income.

Health centers are in all 50 States of the Union.

In conclusion, in administering grants for the health center program, we take great pride in the high evaluation given the program and by the bipartisan support of the Congress, and we fully realize that the program works only as a partnership with those extraordinary local primary care providers providing indispensable, quality clinical service to under-served Americans, their neighbors.

[The prepared statement of Elizabeth M. Duke follows:]

PREPARED STATEMENT OF ELIZABETH M. DUKE, ADMINISTRATOR, HEALTH RESOURCES AND SERVICES ADMINISTRATION

Mr. Chairman, Members of the Subcommittee, thank you for the opportunity to meet with you today on behalf of the Health Resources and Services Administration (HRSA) to discuss the Health Centers Program.

I am so pleased to have the opportunity to address you regarding the Health Centers program. I was here before the Health Subcommittee of the Energy and Commerce Committee on August 1, 2001, to discuss the reauthorization of this program. At that time, the funding for the program was approximately $1.2 billion. We thank you for both your efforts in reauthorizing the program and ensuring funding to expand this worthwhile program to accomplish the President's Initiatives, with a requested FY2006 funding level of approximately $2 billion, a $304 million increase.

Today, I am proud to update you on the success and growth of the program to date. By any measure, we have been enormously successful implementing the President's Health Center Expansion initiative—an effort designed to establish or expand 1,200 health center sites and serve an additional 6.1 million patients annually by the end of 2006. This continues to be a priority because we know that 100 percent of these funds go to provide direct health care services for our neighbors who are most in need.

In 2004, the health center system served an estimated 13.2 million people—about 3 million more than in 2001—at more than 3,650 service delivery sites which represents an increase of more than 600 new and expanded sites since 2001. In 2005, we plan to fund 153 new or expanded health center sites and serve almost 14 million patients.

The President's FY 2006 budget request includes an additional $277 million to complete the President's five-year Health Centers Initiative by increasing the number of health center sites by 275 and significantly expanding 303 existing sites to increase the number of people served by 2.4 million, above 2005 levels, for a total of more than 16.3 million patients.

The President has set a new goal to open a health center or rural health clinic in every poor county that can support one. The Budget includes $26 million to open new health center sites in 40 of the Nation's poorest counties and will support 25 planning grants as well. The goal of the initiative is to leverage the success of the current program to poor counties that can support a Health Center and provide access to primary and preventive health care services particularly in poor communities that are medically underserved.

Health Centers Program

The distinguishing mission of the Health Centers Program is to empower communities to solve their own local access problems and to improve the health status of their underserved and vulnerable populations by building community-based primary care capacity and by offering case management, home visiting, outreach, and other enabling services. The program also addresses significant challenges facing communities by targeting public housing, homeless, and migrant health center development as well. Health Centers provide access to high quality, family oriented, comprehensive primary and preventive health care, regardless of ability to pay.

Health Center grantees, as a result of their receiving from HRSA a grant under section 330 of the Public Health Service (PHS) Act, are eligible for enhanced benefits including Medicaid/Medicare reimbursement, access to the Federal Tort Claims Act (FTCA) program for malpractice coverage and access to the program for discount drugs for patients under section 340B of the PHS Act.

Under the section 330, a Health Center is required to provide primary health services, including those related to family medicine, internal medicine, pediatrics, obstetrics, or gynecology, that are furnished by physicians and where appropriate, physician assistants, nurse practitioners, and nurse midwives. Additional required basic health services include diagnostic laboratory and radiologic services and a series of preventive health services, including prenatal and perinatal services; appropriate cancer screening; well-child services; immunizations against vaccine-preventable diseases; screenings for elevated blood lead levels; communicable diseases and cholesterol; pediatric eye, ear, and dental screenings; voluntary family planning services; and preventive dental services.

Health Centers Requirements

To receive section 330 grant funds, a clinic must meet a number of statutory requirements. The Health Center must: be located in a Federally designated medically underserved area (MUA) or serve a Federally designated medically underserved population (MUP); be a public or private nonprofit health center; provide comprehensive primary health services, referrals, and other services needed to facilitate access to care, such as case management, translation, and transportation; have a governing board, the majority of whose members are patients of the Health Center; provide services to all in the service area regardless of ability to pay; and offer a sliding fee schedule that adjusts according to individual family income.

The requirement that a majority of board members be Health Center patients makes these clinics unique among safety net providers and is designed to ensure that the centers remain responsive to community needs. Under section 330, a Health Center applicant needs to demonstrate the establishment of a governing board that has a 51 percent consumer majority, meets monthly, selects the Health Center's services and hours, approves the Health Center's annual budget, selects the Health Center's director, and establishes the Health Center's general policies.

Health Centers are located in all 50 States, the District of Columbia, and the territories. Currently the Health Center urban-to-rural ratio is even.

Health Centers Awards Process

HRSA accepts, on a competitive basis, applications from eligible organizations seeking a grant for operational support for new and continuing Health Centers. Eligible organizations are public or nonprofit entities including tribal, faith-based and community-based organizations.

The largest category of grant awards includes new access points encompassing both new clinic starts and satellites of existing clinics. Other categories include the expansion of medical capacity at existing locations and new service expansion activities such as enhanced oral health and mental health/substance abuse services.

All eligible and responsive grant applications are referred to an Objective Review Committee (ORC), comprised of experts in the delivery of community health care services, for their independent review and recommendations. When funding decisions are made, each applicant receives a notification letter listing strengths and weaknesses of each section of their application as noted by the ORC. This review approach provides valuable technical assistance for improving future applications for both awardees and those we were not able to approve during a particular cycle due to funding limitations. The process is very competitive and during many cycles, we are able to fund only 20% of the applications submitted. This result reflects a very dynamic program which is encouraging the development of community-based primary health care clinics at a rate greater than we can provide monetary support.

Technical Assistance

HRSA works directly with communities to develop needed resources through the primary care associations in each State. These primary care associations, funded by HRSA, provide ongoing technical assistance involving guidance and options for organizations interested in applying for Health Center grants and to existing Health Center grantees interested in expanding their comprehensive primary care services.

In addition, HRSA assists applicants through grant-writing workshops and other technical assistance activities, which are provided through a contract with the National Association of Community Health Centers. Such activities assist applicants to: demonstrate a high level of need in the community; present a sound proposal to meet this need; show that the organization is ready to rapidly implement the proposal; display responsiveness to the health care environment in the service area; and demonstrate collaborative and coordinated delivery systems for the provision of health care to the underserved in their communities.

Federally-funded health centers are similar to other health care businesses. Like most businesses, at any point in time, approximately 4% of health centers are experiencing significant challenges to their viability. HRSA, with assistance from interdisciplinary teams that may include contractors, grantees and staff, provides intensive technical assistance to grantees to address problems. At all times, continuity of service for the affected population is the first priority under consideration in addressing such challenges.

Health Centers Services

Health Centers offer ambulatory services that reflect the diverse needs of the populations they serve. Because of the combination of low incomes, linguistic barriers, and often poor health status, Health Center patients require access to enabling services as well as comprehensive primary care services.

Health Centers are unique among primary care providers for the array of enabling services they offer, including case management, translation, transportation, outreach, eligibility assistance, and health education. Health Centers commit significant resources to managing chronic conditions including diabetes, asthma, and cardiovascular disease.

In 2003, Health Centers provided more than 49 million encounters, 220,000 mammograms, over 1.4 million pap tests, and 2.27 million encounters for immunizations, as well as nearly 400,000 HIV tests and counseling, perinatal and delivery care for 332,000 women, and translation services to more than 3.5 million patients.

Health Centers are staffed by a combination of clinical, enabling, and administrative personnel. They are typically managed by a chief executive officer and a clinical director. Depending on the size of the patient population, the clinical staff consists of a mixture of primary care physicians, nurse practitioners, physician assistants, substance abuse and mental health specialists, dentists, hygienists, and other health professionals.

Health Centers Financing

Health Centers receive funding from a variety of sources. A majority of Health Centers revenue comes from Federal resources including Medicaid, Medicare, the 330 grant, SCHIP and other Federal programs. On average nationwide, HRSA grants comprise 22 percent of Health Center revenue, but as little as 15 percent depending on the individual community and grant application. At 36 percent, Medicaid is the largest source of revenue for Health Centers, followed by Federal grants. Health Centers serve about 10 percent of all Medicaid enrollees nationally, but in actual Medicaid dollars, this amounts to less than 1 percent of all Medicaid payments to all providers.

For Health Centers(revenues, in addition to Medicaid and the section 330 Federal grant funding, Medicare accounts for 6 percent, self-pay for 6 percent, other third-party payers 9 percent, other State/local government or foundations account for 13 percent and the remaining 6 percent from other sources.

Health Centers Background

The Consolidated Health Centers program has developed over 40 years ago, beginning with the creation of the migrant health center program and followed by the neighborhood health center demonstration projects initiated in 1965 and first funded by Congress as part of the War on Poverty. By the early 1970s, about 100 neighborhood health centers had been established under the Economic Opportunity Act. These centers were designed to provide accessible, dignified personal health services to low-income families. Community and consumer participation in the organization and a patient-majority governing board were features of the Health Center model. With the phase-out of the Office of Economic Opportunity in the early 1970s, the centers supported under this authority were transferred to the Public Health Service. The mandate of the centers was broadened so that comprehensive primary and preventive services were provided to all who came through the doors. The Community Health Center program, as authorized under section 330 of the Public Health Service Act, was established in 1975. A reauthorization that consolidated the separate authorities of the Community, Migrant, Homeless and Public Housing Health Centers under section 330 took place in 1996. Most recently, the Health Care Safety Net Amendments of 2002 reauthorized the Consolidated Health Centers Program through 2006. The 2002 Health Center reauthorization requires that grants be awarded for FY 2002 and beyond in such a way that maintains the proportion of the total appropriation awarded to migrant, homeless and public housing applicants in FY 2001. In general, about 81 percent of funding is awarded to community health centers, with the remaining 19 percent divided across migrant, public housing, and homeless health centers.

Conclusion

Health Centers offer high quality, prevention-oriented, case-managed, family-focused primary care services that result in appropriate and cost-effective use of ambulatory, specialty and in-patient services. Primary care is delivered for all life cycles, and includes a full range of health services. In administering grants for the Health Centers program, we take great pride in the high evaluation given the program, and the bipartisan support of Congress, and fully realize that the program works only as a partnership with those extraordinary local primary care providers providing indispensable quality clinical services to underserved Americans with few health care alternatives.

Mr. WHITFIELD. Thank you, Dr. Duke.

And Mr. Smith, you are recognized for your opening statement.

TESTIMONY OF DENNIS SMITH

Mr. SMITH. Thank you, Mr. Chairman. And thank you, members of the subcommittee, for inviting me today to talk with you all on the role of community health centers as an important part of America's health care system, and in particular, the relationship of the Medicaid and Medicare programs to the CHCs.

I do have a full written statement for the record, and I will try my best not to plow the same ground as the administrator on our points.

But the majority of Medicare and Medicaid dollars that go into the community health centers are through the federally qualified health centers, or FQHCs. Over the years, Medicaid spending has increased substantially. In 1991, Medicaid spending through FQHCs totaled $45 million. Ten years later, Medicaid expenditures in FQHCs had increased to $737 million. Over the last 4 years, spending on FQHCs has nearly doubled to an estimated $1.3 billion. This increased spending is due, in large part, to the President's initiatives to expand community health centers. Medicaid, indeed, is the largest single source of revenues for FQHCs, accounting for 64 percent of patient-related revenues.

Medicare, Medicaid, and SCHIP Benefits Improvement Protection Act of 2000, or BIPA, established a prospective payment system for FQHCs. This system, which has been in place since January 2001, replaced the previous cost-based reimbursement system for health centers under Medicaid. The prospective payment system establishes a per-visit payment rate for each FQHC in advance. And since fiscal year 2002, payments made under this system have been adjusted annually for inflation using the Medicare Economic Index.

States have the option of using an alternative payment mechanism, provided that the payment rate is not lower than what would have been paid under the new PPS. States have made a variety of choices in how they want to set their reimbursement rates—which system to use, the PPS or alternative methodologies. I think it is very important to emphasize that the FQHCs themselves must agree to the alternative methodologies.

In addition, States are required to make supplemental payments to FQHCs that provide care to Medicaid beneficiaries when they are enrolled in a managed care plan to cover the difference between the rates paid by managed care plans and the FQHC's prospective payment rate. So again, Congress has been very clear that FQHC's are an important part of the delivery system. We want to make certain that those payments make the FQHCs whole for the cost that they provide to beneficiaries.

Very briefly, in addition to Medicaid expenditures, Medicare spends $265 million on services provided through FQHCs. The Medicare reimbursement rate is based on an all-inclusive per-visit payment amount based on reasonable costs as determined through filing of a Medicare cost report. These are subject to one of two upper payment limits, not the other upper payment limits that we often discuss, but its own upper payment limit, depending on whether the FQHC is located in an urban or a rural area. For calendar year 2005, the upper payment limit is $109.88 for urban centers, $94.48 for rural centers.

In conclusion, community health centers are an important part of the Medicare and Medicaid network of providers. Substantial growth in expenditures reflects the increase in access to care at CHCs through President Bush's initiatives as well as through the partnerships that have been formed over the years between HRSA, CMS, the centers, the States, and the managed care organizations.

I look forward to addressing the questions that you might have, and thank you, again, for the opportunity to appear before you today.

[The prepared statement of Dennis Smith follows:]

PREPARED STATEMENT OF DENNIS SMITH, DIRECTOR, CENTER FOR MEDICAID AND STATE OPERATIONS, CENTERS FOR MEDICARE AND MEDICAID SERVICES

Chairman Whitfield, Congressman Stupak, thank you for inviting me to testify on the role of the Medicaid program in serving millions of Americans who seek care through community health centers (CHCs). CHCs are an important part of America's health care safety net, providing comprehensive primary and preventive health care services to all who seek care. They serve in rural areas or in inner-city neighborhoods, places where too many people do not have the access to the quality health care they require. CHCs exist in areas where economic, geographic, or cultural barriers limit access to primary health care for a substantial portion of the population; and, they tailor services to the needs of the community. Services include primary and preventive health care, prenatal services, dental care, and essential ancillary services such as laboratory tests, X-ray, environmental health, and pharmacy services. In addition, they provide services such as outreach and health education, transportation, and translation services.

CHCS, STATE MEDICAID PROGRAMS, AND MEDICARE SERVE AMERICANS WITH LIMITED INCOMES

The majority of Medicare and Medicaid dollars that go into CHCs are through the Federally Qualified Health Centers (FQHCs). Congress established the FQHC program in 1989 to respond to concerns that health centers were using grant funds intended to support care for the uninsured to supplement Medicare and Medicaid payments. FQHCs under Medicare and Medicaid include three types of centers:

- Community health centers that receive grants under section 330 of the Public Health Service Act;
- FQHC "look-alikes"—centers that meet all of requirements for a community health center under section 330 of the Public Health Service Act, but do not receive such a grant, and that are not owned, controlled or operated by another entity; and
- Outpatient health programs or tribal facilities operated by a tribe or tribal facility under the Indian Self-Determination Act or by an urban Indian organization receiving funds under Title V of the Indian Health Care Improvement Act for the provision of primary health services.

Over the years, Medicaid spending through FQHCs has increased substantially. As recently as 1991, Federal Medicaid spending on services provided to Medicaid beneficiaries by FQHCs totaled $45 million. Federal Medicaid expenditures in FQHCs have increased since then to $778 million in FY 2004. This increased spending is due in large part to an increase of about 500 new health center sites under the President's health center initiative. (These figures do not include expenditures through managed care contracts or the state share of Medicaid funding). Total Federal and State Medicaid spending total $1.3 billion in FY 2004.

According to HRSA, Medicaid is the largest single source of revenue for the FQHCs. Medicaid accounts for 36 percent of total revenue of the FQHCs.

CMS designates FQHC look-alikes based on the recommendation of HRSA. When CMS receives a recommendation from HRSA, CMS notifies the State Medicaid agency of a pending application for FQHC designation and provides the state with an opportunity to comment on the application. Once all issues are addressed, CMS notifies HRSA and the State Medicaid agency that the application has been approved and HRSA notifies the center of the approval. In CY 2004, CMS approved 26 applications. Currently, six applications are under review.

MEDICAID COVERS FQHCS AS A MANDATORY BENEFIT

As mentioned earlier, FQHCs provide a package of primary and preventive care services to Medicaid beneficiaries. These services include physician, nurse practitioner, physician assistant, clinical psychologist and clinical social worker, plus any other ambulatory service that is covered in the state plan. FQHCs are paid under the Medicaid program for services on a per visit basis, rather than billing separately for each service provided when a patient visits a health center.

The Medicare, Medicaid, and SCHIP Benefits Improvement and Protection Act of 2000 (BIPA) established a prospective payment system for FQHCs. This system, which has been in place since January 2001, replaced the previous cost-based reimbursement system for health centers under Medicaid. The prospective payment system establishes a per visit payment rate for each FQHC in advance. The 2001 payment rate was based on the average of each FQHC's reasonable costs per visit in FY 1999 and FY 2000. Since FY 2002, payments made under this system have been adjusted annually for inflation using the Medicare Economic Index. Payments also are adjusted based on increases or decreases in change in scope of services provided.

States have the option of using an alternative payment mechanism, provided the payment rate is not lower than what would be paid under the new PPS. For example, states may opt to establish an alternative PPS or retain the original cost-based reimbursement system. CMS must review and approve the payment system; and, the FQHC must agree to the alternative methodology. Most states are using the PPS option established under BIPA, while 15 states opted to use cost-based reimbursement and eight states elected to implement an alternative PPS to pay at least a portion of their FQHC costs.

In addition, states are required to make supplemental payments to FQHCs that provide care to Medicaid beneficiaries enrolled in a managed care plan to cover the difference between the rates paid by managed care plans and the FQHC's prospective payment rate. FQHCs receive the same payment rate from managed care plans that the plans pay to other providers for similar services. This supplemental payment provision was added as an incentive to FQHCs to participate in managed care plans. FQHCs are guaranteed a PPS rate as a minimum to participate in a managed care plan.

MEDICARE PAYMENTS BASED ON REASONABLE COSTS

FQHC services also are available to Medicare beneficiaries under Part B. The Medicare FQHC benefit provides coverage for a full range of primary care services (and services incident thereto) including physician, physician assistant, nurse practitioner, and certain other non-physician practitioner services such as clinical social worker and clinical psychologist services. The benefit also covers a range of preventive services as well as pneumococal and influenza vaccines. In CY 2003, almost 900,000 Medicare beneficiaries received care at a section 330-funded FQHC.

Medicare pays FQHCs an all-inclusive per visit payment amount, based on reasonable costs as determined through the filing of its Medicare cost report. The FQHC's all-inclusive per visit payment amount is subject to one of two upper payment limits (UPL), depending upon whether the FQHC is located in an urban or rural area. In CY 2005, the UPL is $109.88 for urban centers and $94.48 for rural centers. In FY 2004, Medicare spent about $265 million on services provided by FQHCs. To ensure payment rates are appropriate, CMS and HRSA are jointly evaluating the current UPLs for Medicare FQHC services.

In addition, the Medicare Prescription Drug, Improvement, and Modernization Act of 2003 (MMA) establishes a wrap-around payment in Medicare, similar to the supplemental payment in Medicaid. CMS will pay FQHCs the difference between what a Medicare Advantage health care plan pays the FQHC, and the reasonable cost payments the FQHC otherwise would receive under Medicare fee-for-service. Medicare Advantage plans must pay FQHCs the same levels and amounts they pay other providers for similar services. This provision becomes effective for services provided on or after January 1, 2006 and contract years beginning on or after January 1, 2006.

ENSURING FQHCS PARTICIPATE IN THE MEDICARE PRESCRIPTION DRUG PROGRAM

HRSA and CMS have been working closely together on efforts to implement the new prescription drug benefit under Medicare Part D, and will be working to make sure health centers are a key part of that effort, particularly with respect to outreach and education of low-income Medicare beneficiaries who are eligible for the low-income subsidy program and will be eligible for a comprehensive drug benefit with minimal copayments. Also, health centers with pharmacies will be able to participate in prescription drug coverage plans and Medicare Health Plans with prescription drug coverage. In addition, the final rule implementing the MMA provides that prescription drug coverage plans and Medicare Health Plans may count FQHC pharmacies in meeting the MMA pharmacy access standards, and this will give these plans incentives to include FQHC pharmacies in their plan networks.

CONCLUSION

CHCs are an important part of the Medicare and Medicaid networks of providers. The substantial growth in expenditures reflects the increase in access to care at CHCs through the President's initiative as well as partnerships that have been formed over the years between HRSA, CMS, the Centers, the states, and managed care organizations.

Thank you again for this opportunity and I look forward to answering any questions you might have.

Mr. WHITFIELD. Well, thank you all very much for your testimony. We appreciate your taking the time to be with us, as I indicated.

And Dr. Duke, I will begin the question period here.

And you mentioned in your testimony that one of your goals is to be sure that 40 of the Nation's poorest counties each has a community health center located within their boundaries. How many of those 40 counties have a community health center today?

Ms. DUKE. The initiative, as the President described it, is to target high-poverty counties that have no health center or rural health clinic in them today.

Mr. WHITFIELD. This 40 figure that you mentioned, so you are talking about areas that do not have a center already?

Ms. DUKE. Yes, sir; that is correct.

Mr. WHITFIELD. I thought that you were talking about that it was an overall goal to be sure that the 40 poorest counties had a center and that some of them already did have a center, but that is not what you are talking about.

Ms. DUKE. No, sir. The idea is that there are many, many counties that do not have a rural health clinic or an FQHC.

Mr. WHITFIELD. Right.

Ms. DUKE. And the goal would be to allow competition to increase the number of poor counties that have a center.

Mr. WHITFIELD. Well, what role do States play in winning these 330 grants? And I ask that question, because is there any concern that some States just may be more adept at this than others? I noticed, for example, that Alaska has, like, 21 grantees, and they have a population of about 670,000. A State like Kentucky, and I just happen to be from Kentucky, has 4.5 million and we have 12. So do States play an important role in being successful in the awarding of these grants?

Ms. DUKE. The process by which these get awarded, perhaps if I could talk about the process and then talk about the State role in that, would that be helpful?

Mr. WHITFIELD. Yes. Right.

Ms. DUKE. The process under which grants are awarded is a competitive process. And the requirements are that to be awarded a health center, it must be in a medically under-served area——

Mr. WHITFIELD. Right.

Ms. DUKE. [continuing] and that it must be a non-for-profit or a public entity. And it is competitive. And it has been a very competitive process. We receive far more applications than we have capacity to fund. And the States do get engaged in this activity, because we have initiated a strategic planning process. And the primary care associations in each State work to identify needs for health centers and provide technical assistance to communities in building the foundation to be actually able to compete. And some have been very, very engaged in that process and others have been, perhaps, less engaged.

But interesting, you can actually see the results of the way that activity has gone in the sense that intensive strategic planning has produced increased numbers of awards to States over the last 4 to 5 years.

Mr. WHITFIELD. And what are some of the States that are most adept at that?

Ms. DUKE. Well, I think the one that I took particular attention to in the recent competition was Texas, which had a high uninsured rate where the Primary Care Association and the legislature put together a strategic plan, and in the last competition, they achieved 10 health center awards in that last competition.

Mr. WHITFIELD. And how many were granted nationwide?

Ms. DUKE. In that round, I think it was 88.

Mr. WHITFIELD. So Texas received 10 of those?

Ms. DUKE. Eighty-eight plus seventeen. I am sorry. It is 88 plus 17.

Mr. WHITFIELD. Okay. Now the Objective Review Committee, who is a member of the Objective Review Committee, and how is it decided who is a member of that committee?

Ms. DUKE. Objective Review Committees are selected from people who have expertise in community health delivery. And it is our goal to have the members of the Objective Review Committees cycle on and off so we don't have the same people on all of the time. We have made a very aggressive campaign to have more and more people involved in that process. We think it is educational for them, and it certainly provides fairness for the community. And we receive about 100 applications a month for people to enter the ranks of serving on these objective review panels.

So it is a widely diverse group.

Mr. WHITFIELD. And is there a set number of members on that Objective Review Committee?

Ms. DUKE. It is not a set number, but the goal is to have a sufficient number that there can be dialog that they can carry on the weight of the number of applications, because we get hundreds of applications, and we break them down into a certain number per panel. So they work very hard, and they do a great deal of work, because each of these applications is about 80 pages long.

Mr. WHITFIELD. So do you appoint them, or who appoints them?

Ms. DUKE. I do not touch them. They are basically taken care of in the routine process of our centralized grants management process. We have a centralized grants management process that sets up the Objective Review Committees. That is to say it is separate from the program office that runs the health center program. And it is separate from my office. It is set up by people who do professionally grant administration. And they are set up objectively, and then they have a scoring process that is designed to get around the problem, which is inherent in human nature, and, as we used to say in the school world, some people are easy graders and some people are hard graders, and so they set up a process to distinguish out the outliners so that a fair score——

Mr. WHITFIELD. But they don't make the final decision?

Ms. DUKE. No, sir; they don't make the final decision, but their weighting is very significant.

Mr. WHITFIELD. Okay.

Ms. DUKE. The final decision has to rest on addressing other issues, like their financial viability.

Mr. WHITFIELD. I read an article for this hearing, and it may have been somebody's testimony, I can't remember right now, but it said that last year, 106 million visits were made to hospital emergency rooms and that 58 percent of those really were not necessary, it was not proper to be at a hospital, and maybe going to a community health center would have been better. Are you familiar with that statistic? And has your agency conducted any studies on the relationship of savings by these community health centers for hospital emergency rooms, for example? Any sort of study like that that you conducted?

Ms. DUKE. Sir, I could give you two. I am not familiar with that particular statistic, but we could provide copies for you, I am familiar with the results of one study that indicated that by having patients have a medical home at a health center, that that drives down the inappropriate hospitalizations by about 11 percent and drives down inappropriate use of emergency rooms by 19 percent. And we could provide that for you. The other thing is that we have seen some communities that have come together to compete for health center programs who have then networked themselves together with the community health centers and hospitals and private physicians and so forth to address this question of the inappropriate use of very expensive emergency room care. And we have seen in one instance where we provided a grant for 3 years to support that kind of networking, and at the end of the 3 years, the community sustained that approach with the view that they were saving enough in the hospitals' emergency rooms to support the networking costs associated with it.

So it is a good investment.

Mr. WHITFIELD. Have you had any experience with a small hospital, say a small rural hospital, that is a critical access hospital, as an example, that was having such financial difficulty that they decided they wanted to convert to become a community health center with emphasis on primary care and preventative care? Are you aware of an example of that happening anywhere in the country?

Ms. DUKE. I don't have a specific instance in mind, but that is one of the things that we have seen is where hospitals previously had run outpatient clinics and ultimately decided to give up that line and a community board took over the outpatient work and ultimately competed for and won a grant as a federally supported FQHC.

Mr. WHITFIELD. Well, my time is expired, and I recognize the gentleman from Michigan.

Ms. DUKE. Thank you, sir.

Mr. STUPAK. Thank you, Mr. Chairman, and welcome to our witnesses.

Ms. DUKE. Thank you.

Mr. STUPAK. Mr. Smith, if I may ask you a question on Medicaid here. The large Medicaid cuts are particularly hurting our rural areas, as folks in rural areas are more likely to receive Medicaid and to be uninsured, and 30 percent of the children in rural areas have Medicaid or SCHIP coverage compared to 19 percent in urban areas. Nearly 25 percent of residents in rural counties are uninsured.

In my statement, I mentioned Michigan and how our unemployment is at 7.5 percent and our demand on Medicaid is unprecedented. We are covering a lot of people who are employed. We have a job and can't afford insurance. So our question is, we are having all of these people on here. We have cuts coming to Medicaid. Where does Michigan go? Actually one out of every four people now in Michigan are on Medicaid. So who do we dump in Michigan if we don't have the funds to take care of it? If you take a look at our Medicaid in Michigan, it has gone up 30 percent but yet we have held our costs to less than 5 percent. So I think Michigan has really done a good job, but we are just at the point now where we have to start making tough choices. So who do we dump? The senior in the nursing homes? The children with disabilities? Or cut providers?

Mr. SMITH. We are very pleased with the partnership we have had with Michigan over the past several years. We have helped Michigan expand health insurance coverage through the HIFA waiver. We helped Michigan come up with one of the most innovative cost containment proposals in the country by starting the drug purchasing arrangements. Michigan was the originator, but it has expanded to other States as well.

Mr. STUPAK. Sure, but under that program, we are getting penalized for being efficient.

Mr. SMITH. I think that what we are finding in Michigan, and other States as well, States are reconsidering new ways to deliver services in more cost effective and innovative ways, including in long-term care settings. A third of Medicaid's spending is on long-term care. We are seeing States move more into home and community-based services, expanding services for people to stay in their own homes rather than go into institutional care. We think this is part of the solution.

Mr. STUPAK. Well, let me ask the question this way. Medicaid was set up so that when unemployment goes up, Medicaid would be there to take care of those people who lost their insurance or can't afford it anymore. But yet what we are seeing in Michigan, more and more people are going on Medicaid, and our reimbursement, or help from the Federal Government, has decreased, the exact opposite of the way it was supposed to be when the program was passed by Congress. So how can we justify increased caseloads in Michigan but yet less money? Something has got to give. Who don't we cover any more?

Mr. SMITH. In large part, when people become uninsured, they are not eligible for Medicaid in the first place. For example, if you are an unemployed single male, you are not going to become eligible for Medicaid.

Mr. STUPAK. But a lot of these are not unemployed single males.

Let me ask you this question. The Energy and Commerce Committee has been directed to find $15 to $20 billion in cuts over the next 5 years. If you take a look at it, the President's proposed Medicaid cuts, it is probably $8 billion, but yet in the budget resolution, we are directed to come up with $15 to $16 to $20 billion in cuts, and we have this commission. Can you provide some specific ways Congress could cut funding to Medicaid that were not included in the President's budget proposal that CBO scored at $8 billion? And this commission that is set up, wouldn't it be better if we had them look outside the budget process on ways we can save money as opposed to looking within the Federal budget process?

Mr. SMITH. I think that the President's budget provides a lot of guidance for how we think you can lower the rate of growth in the Medicaid program. Medicaid over the next 10 years is going to spend $5 trillion. And you mentioned Michigan's rate of growth of being around 5 percent. In fact, Michigan has been holding their rate of growth to below the national average for each of the 5 years. So we know that States can adopt ways to lower their rate of growth of spending and still deliver quality services and, in the case of Michigan, expand coverage as well. What we have——

Mr. STUPAK. But rate of growth, to make sure we are on the same page here, are you talking about spending, sir?

Mr. SMITH. Yes, Mr. Stupak.

Mr. STUPAK. Well, I am talking about rate of growth to increase the people we have on here. I agree, the spending is down, but the number of people on it are going up.

Mr. SMITH. And as I said, and you stated as well, Michigan's rate of growth is around 5 percent.

Mr. STUPAK. Correct.

Mr. SMITH. That is lower than the national rate of growth.

Mr. STUPAK. And they have cut every possible way to keep that less than 5 percent. They even came up with a new drug program, and yet we are being penalized by the Federal Government for doing that. We are going to lose money underneath the program reimbursement. So how do we do it? I mean, I am not wrong in my theory on why we have Medicaid, so when unemployment goes up, Medicaid is supposed to go up and be there to take care of the unemployed. When unemployment goes down, Medicaid should go down, right? That is the theory behind the program.

Mr. SMITH. And that is the essential partnership that still exists in the Medicaid program as well.

Mr. STUPAK. The partnership exists, but the reimbursement isn't there.

Mr. SMITH. The Federal dollars follow State dollars, and the States make the decisions beyond the Federal requirements of eligibility and services. The States are the ones making the decisions on who to cover, what services——

Mr. STUPAK. But unlike the Federal Government, the States have to balance their budget. The Federal Government does not. And Michigan, as it balances its budget, is balancing a budget, especially when we come to Medicaid when $1 out of every $4 is on Medicaid, is either on seniors, on nursing homes, disabled people, or the unemployed.

Let me just leave you with this thought. Hopefully this commission will look at ways to modernize Medicaid outside the budget process. I would hope you would encourage them to do that. I would just look within this Federal budget, because I think there are other ways of doing it, and Michigan would be one good example, if you would take a look at it.

Let me ask Dr. Duke this question.

You said in your opening, and I found it pretty fascinating, that about 2001 we had 10 million people on the system, and your goal is to get, by the end of fiscal year 2005, 16.3 million. You know, we are putting more people on, but the reimbursement isn't there, and you are bringing on new centers and the centers now, as we will hear in the next panel, don't have enough money to compete. So for putting on 60 percent more people than we did 5 years ago, we have more health centers than we had 5 years ago, but we are not keeping up with the reimbursement rates from the Federal Government the same, so again, something has got to give. Either we have got to cut back on providers, we have got to cut back on the existing ones. We are going to have to find money elsewhere, correct?

Ms. DUKE. The health centers are supported by a variety of funding sources. The grants under the Public Health Service Act constitute about 22 percent of their funding. Medicaid is about a third of their funding. But they also have funding that comes in from the State and from private philanthropy, and in fact, about 75 percent of their funding does not come through the program that we conduct. They are locally funded as well. So I don't want to just tie the public health centers to one source of funding.

Mr. STUPAK. Sure. Well, let me ask it this way. From just the Federal Government, if you had 10 million people being served, and I don't know how many centers there were back in 2001, but you had it in your testimony——

Ms. DUKE. 3,200.

Mr. STUPAK. 3,200. And in 2006, you are going to have how many?

Ms. DUKE. 4,400.

Mr. STUPAK. Okay. Are the 3,200 going to get the same amount of money in real dollars, not taking into account inflation, what they got in 2001? Will they get that same amount in 2006?

Ms. DUKE. Well, there will be a different body of health centers.

Mr. STUPAK. Sure. We are expanding them.

Ms. DUKE. There will be a different body of health centers, and they will have different sources of funding. They will have Medicaid. They will have our grant. They will have Medicare. They will have private philanthropy——

Mr. STUPAK. Well, that is the same thing they had in 2001. The point being, how can we continue to expand a program if we are not taking care of existing health centers now?

Ms. DUKE. The health centers now have received, over the last several years, grant money, and they have received base adjustments, $31 million in 2005. In addition, they receive sources of funding outside of the Federal Government.

Mr. STUPAK. I agree with all of that. The Rural Flexibility Grant Program, it is a great program. Let us zero it out this year. How do we justify that? How about the Rural Health Reach Grant Program? That is $28 million. It took a 70 percent cut this year. So I mean, how do we make that stuff up?

Ms. DUKE. The Rural Health Program is funded under a different category, and the——

Mr. STUPAK. Or not funded. But go ahead.

Ms. DUKE. The reasoning behind that has been that the rural areas are significantly benefited, about $25 billion, under the Medicare Modernization Act, and the categorical programs that were under our program were considered to be now not needed since the funding would come through MMA.

Mr. STUPAK. Do you really think any of the health care centers are going to say we no longer need the Rural Flexibility Grant Program or the rural outreach grants, that they are no longer needed underneath your program? They still need those programs, don't they?

Ms. DUKE. The rural health centers and the variety of recipients of those grants are in the process of just getting used to the new act that is just coming into implementation.

Mr. STUPAK. Getting used to no money? I mean, if you zeroed out the program, they are just getting used to it.

Ms. DUKE. The new act will come in in 2006, and that is the 2006 budget you are quoting.

Mr. STUPAK. Right. Okay.

Mr. WALDEN [presiding]. The Chair now recognizes the chairman of the full committee, Mr. Barton, for questions.

Chairman BARTON. Thank you.

And I don't think I will take 10 minutes.

First, Dr. Duke, I want to thank you for your assistance in helping make the decision to fund the health clinic in Tarrant County at John Peter Smith. We appreciate that.

I guess my basic question is just kind of a general one. How many counties and cities do we have that could use a rural health clinic or a public health clinic that don't have them right now? What percent of the truly eligible needy population is not being served that could be served? Are we serving half of the population, two-thirds of the population, a fourth of the population?

Ms. DUKE. Sir, I don't have an exact number to give you there. We have a number of counties that have significant populations at below 200 percent of poverty. The question is some of them have a rural health clinic. Some of them have an FQHC, so I don't exactly have the exact number to give you at this moment.

Chairman BARTON. Well, but give me some number. I mean, how close are we to saying that we are generally meeting the need that the program was designed to meet? I am not holding you to any specificity, just generically. Are we——

Ms. DUKE. I will just use the data I have myself. If I go by the number of applications we receive versus the number of applications are we are actually able to fund, that might be a piece of data. We can fund about 20 percent of the grant applications we receive, which means that four-fifths of those that we receive, we can't fund.

Chairman BARTON. And so all of those are qualified? They are legitimate applications that meet the minimum requirements?

Ms. DUKE. Yes, all of the grants that I am referring to there were deemed to be eligible to compete and had applications that could be reviewed by an objective review committee.

Chairman BARTON. Okay. So just kind of generally, we are only meeting 20 percent, or one out of five, and it could be 1 out of 4 or 1 out of 3, but we can't say that we are meeting 7 out of 10. We are not at 70 percent or 80 percent. We are under 50 percent, not over 50 percent.

Ms. DUKE. We have a base of 3,200 that we started with in 2001, and so given that as a base, which lays a foundation, then on top of that, the competition is that we are funding about one-fifth of our applications.

Chairman BARTON. Okay. This application process, I mean, I am familiar with it now, because I went through it in my home county in my home District, do you consider that to be a fair application process?

Ms. DUKE. Yes, it is a fair application process. It has many, many challenges. One of the challenges is ascertaining need. Need exists in a variety of ways as you go across this really very diverse, vast country. And need looks different in Alaska than it looks in Florida. It looks different in Montana than in Texas. And one of the things we did fairly early on was to change the process to allow communities to tell us what need looked like in their community and then tell us how they were going to meet that need. And that need boils down to what are the barriers to care in the area and what are the disparities and health results that come from those barriers? So we have just put on a Federal Register notice, and we have received some answers back that we are in the process of having the experts review. To get feedback from the communities as to the adequacy of those criteria and also the percentage of weight that should be put on need in both the first round of scoring, which is just strictly on need, and then in the second round, the percentage of need as related to how that need is going to be met.

So we are constantly trying to assess that process, make sure that it is fair, and make sure that it is getting a return of good health care for the investment the taxpayers are making.

Chairman BARTON. My last question, Mr. Chairman, and I will refer to this to Mr. Smith.

We are looking at Medicaid reconciliation and Medicaid reform. We are going to do that in our Health Subcommittee later this summer. Are these federally qualified health centers an avenue that could be utilized more to get better quality care for low income at a competitive price if we were to make a few changes in the current Medicaid laws?

Mr. SMITH. Mr. Chairman, I think that FQHCs in particular are vitally important because of access in under-served areas, and they are very important for that. In terms of reform or generating a lower rate of growth——

Chairman BARTON. No, I am talking about expanding them, not contracting them, by taking the pressure off emergency rooms in our central hospitals, could we get better quality at less cost if we expanded the use of these federally qualified health centers? That is probably a better way to phrase the question.

Mr. SMITH. I think they are key players in under-served areas. In terms of great impact on the overall program, as I said, Medicaid reimbursement for FQHCs is about $1.3 billion out of total Medicaid spending of well over $300 billion. They are very important for local areas in giving access, but nationally, FQHCs are a relatively small part of the program.

Chairman BARTON. I am going to yield back. I yield to Mr. Walden.

Mr. WALDEN. Thank you, Mr. Chairman.

I was just going to point out that as we have this discussion about the size of the budget for the federally qualified centers versus overall Medicaid, it is important to go back to a comment made earlier and the work that is being done to look at the savings that are achieved for Medicaid because we have these centers in place. And it was pointed out to me that a 1980 study looked at a set of Medicaid patients who used community health centers back then and had a 30 to 65 percent lower hospitalization rate and used 12 percent to 48 percent less total Medicaid funds than a similar group of Medicaid patients who did not use such centers.

So if these data hold true today, 25 years later or 20 years later, whatever it is, they are enormous savings. I mean, it is just sort of logical that if you are not feeling well and you can go to a health center in your community and get checked out and sort of do the preventive end of things, you would probably be more likely to do that, at least in this period of time, than waiting if there is no clinic. That means I have got to go to the hospital, and you wait and suddenly you just go to the ER. And the most expensive portal of health care is open to you. And so it just seems to me, logically, that if we could encourage families and encourage these health care clinics——

Chairman BARTON. Especially if only 20 percent of the eligible population has one of these.

Mr. WALDEN. Yes. And that is why I think the President is on track.

Chairman BARTON. Expand this program and——

Mr. WHITFIELD. I might add, Mr. Chairman, that I have heard some people make a comment, half seriously and half not seriously, that we might be better of as a Nation, from a health care perspective, if say half of the money spent on Medicaid now was used to create additional community health care centers, that that would be a greater savings, provide better health care, in other words think outside the box a new model.

Chairman BARTON. Isn't it great to have these hearings so we can talk to each other while you all watch?

Mr. WALDEN. Well, can I just finish up on——

Chairman BARTON. Sure. I am going to yield the balance of my time to Congressman Walden, the vice-chairman of the subcommittee.

Mr. WALDEN. Thank you. I appreciate that, Mr. Chairman.

There is one question. I noticed today, in the Congress Daily, Mr. Smith, you are quoted talking about——

Chairman BARTON. This just means after he asks his questions he can leave. He doesn't have to wait for another hour. That is how sneaky he is.

Mr. WALDEN. Well, because I had to yield, when I was in the chair, to you, because you are like senior and all and have the big gavel.

So in the 43 seconds I have left on your time, I guess the question is as we look for savings, one of the things that has been identified recently is some pharmaceuticals that are given to certain people, and specifically when it comes to things like Viagra, for potential sex offenders through Medicaid. You have spoken out on that. I mean, are there other things like that that we need to be looking at when we look at how to direct the money to the best place?

Mr. SMITH. I think there are lots of areas in Medicaid to look at. FQHCs show that when you have access, it is going to lower costs for the total part of the system. We have talked, and Chairman Barton held a hearing last December on how Medicaid is overpaying for prescription drugs, finding ways for Medicaid to be a better payer, and the extent to which Medicaid can get to the under-utilization and the over-utilization by improving service delivery. I think that is where the promise really lies. And we have seniors who are on drugs that are contraindicated for them individually. You go to a PACE program and when I go in, I inevitably ask, "What is the average number of drugs a senior is on when they come into the clinic?" Once they have started, 6 months later, they are on half of the number of drugs they were on when they started. So I think there is a lot of over-utilization in the program and by improving the way we deliver services we will also improve health care and lower the rate of growth.

Mr. WALDEN. Well, the figure on these impotence drugs are like $2 billion for Medicare and Medicaid combined. So we are talking about billions around here. It adds up.

Mr. SMITH. Yes, sir.

Mr. WHITFIELD. The gentleman's time has expired.

I might also just add that I had, myself, asked the General Accounting Office to do a little more comprehensive study of some of the savings to Medicaid and Medicare as a result of having these community health centers, which touched on some issues that Chairman Barton raised, and I am looking forward to their getting back with us on that study.

At this time, I will recognize the gentlelady from Wisconsin, Ms. Baldwin.

Ms. BALDWIN. Thank you, Mr. Chairman.

My question is for Dr. Duke. I would like to get your opinions on the sparsely populated area preference, which has been in effect since 1995. And it is a provision that I would say adversely affects my State, and as I understand, most States in the Midwest, East, and South of our country.

Now let me just go through my understanding of this preference before I ask your opinion.

My understanding is that a sparsely populated area is a preference, which is unlike a priority designation, and that a priority designation can add a few points to an applicant's score, but a preference requires that an application that meets minimal qualifications must be funded ahead of other applicants, perhaps with significantly higher overall scores. Thus, many sparsely populated area applicants that meet the needs test cutoff and score well enough to be fundable are allowed to really jump to the front of the funding line, regardless of their overall comparative merit and score.

I represent part of the State of Wisconsin and much of Wisconsin is quite rural. But none of the counties in Wisconsin meet the very narrow criteria to be a sparsely populated area, which, to my understanding, is a county with a population of seven persons or fewer per square mile.

I think you previously testified that a few years back, in 2002, over $13 million was provided to 24 sparsely populated applicants in eight States, yet 125 non-sparsely populated applicants with higher scores than the lowest scoring sparsely populated applicant were passed over for funding.

So I guess I would ask whether you would be supportive of Congress making the sparsely populated applicants a priority rather than a preference. And I would also be interested in knowing what changes in the scoring process you would support in order to make sure that rural applicants get their fair share of these grants.

Ms. DUKE. The legislation, as you describe it, sets up certain categories of applicants, among them sparsely populated, which, as you describe, is a requirement that has a population number of seven——

Ms. BALDWIN. Seven people or fewer per square mile.

Ms. DUKE. [continuing] people or fewer per square mile, and certain States fit that requirement.

One of the barriers to care that is part of the consideration is the issue of geography and distance. And that was the comment I made a bit back that America is an incredibly diverse country. And so the barriers to care in one State may look significantly different from the barriers to care in another State or in a section of a State. So that was the thinking of the Congress in putting that sparsely populated provision in. There are also provisions for special treatment of migrant health centers, public housing, and homeless health centers as well. And the justification is, as I have indicated, the administration does not have a position on changing those designations at this point, but I will raise the issue.

Ms. BALDWIN. Okay. And then for Mr. Smith, I am certainly very supportive of the increases in funding for community health centers. And in my State, centers have been able to use additional funding to expand. In conversations with some of the directors, it is my impression that CMS and HRSA have put a large emphasis, and perhaps even a requirement, on build-out. For example, if a clinic is expanding, they must also build dental suites as part of that expansion. But what happens, it seems that less emphasis is given to funding the actual health care that would be provided in these build-outs. So I guess my question is what kind of requirements are placed on centers that are expanding? And is it appropriate to place such emphasis on build-outs without a corresponding emphasis on the services delivered?

Mr. SMITH. I thank you for the question, but I think actually the administrator would be better able to respond on build-out.

Ms. DUKE. I will have to get back to you for the record on that. I need to check out what that issue is.

Ms. BALDWIN. Okay.

Ms. DUKE. I apologize. I need to follow up on that.

Ms. BALDWIN. We would be happy to work with you to get some more information.

Ms. DUKE. Okay.

Ms. BALDWIN. I do not have any further questions, and I would yield back the remainder of my time.

Mr. WHITFIELD. Thank you, Ms. Baldwin.

At this time, we would recognize Mr. Walden.

Mr. WALDEN. Yes. Mr. Chairman, I had a couple minutes of the other chair's time, and I know we have got votes coming up, so I will yield to other members.

Mr. WHITFIELD. Okay. Mr. Burgess, you are recognized.

Mr. BURGESS. Thank you, Mr. Chairman.

I will, too, try to condense this because of votes.

Dr. Duke, thank you for your commitment, the administration's commitment to the community health centers program, and thanks for your interest to work with Congress to continue the expansion currently underway. The need for the comprehensive services that these centers provide is on the rise, based on the number of applications that your office receives annually. And I see this need back home, where I am very eager to have another health center established in Tarrant County. Chairman Barton correctly pointed out that one was placed in North Fort Worth just recently, but we very badly need one in the southeast part of town.

Can you tell me how many applications you received last year that were acceptable for funding? If there were no limits on funding, how many would you have funded?

Ms. DUKE. I think I am just going to have to report on one round. I believe we received 330 some in the round, and we were able to fund 76, I think, in that round, and it came back to about 25 percent. But that is from memory. And what I would rather do, frankly, is to share with you a table that would have the accurate data rather than trying to do it from memory.

Mr. BURGESS. Very well. If additional funding is coming your way, what plans do you have for ensuring that the maximum number of proposals are going to be accepted to receive funding?

Ms. DUKE. We have put together a strategic planning process in each State that is led by the primary care association in each State to identify where needs are and to give technical assistance to communities to build those areas. What we are doing right now is those plans are developed and the applications that are coming in are extraordinarily good. Basically, we follow the legislation, as I just mentioned to Ms. Baldwin, and we follow the requirements for the set-asides for the various categories. And then we take the available money and we fund centers in order of their scores until we have no more money. And so we have lots of applications that are high-quality applications that we would continue to fund and we believe that the strategic planning process will continue to bring in good applications from deserving communities.

Mr. BURGESS. Very well. Thank you.

Mr. Smith, if I understand this correctly, Medicaid reimbursement at a federally qualified health center or a look-alike facility, is at the usual and customary rate as opposed to the Medicare maximum allowable, is that correct?

Mr. SMITH. There are a couple of different ways. The payment methodologies can use a prospective payment system or a cost-reimbursement system that is then indexed, or an alternative that the FQHCs and the States can agree upon. So there are really about three different ways you could potentially pay. And then on top of that, if you are serving an individual in Medicaid who is enrolled in managed care, the managed care plan may be the payer, but the State would also pay a supplemental rate at an FQHC site in order to make the FQHC whole.

Mr. BURGESS. Well, certainly I support the administration's goal of providing more federally qualified health centers. Given the chairman's discussion and Mr. Walden's discussion, I just can't help but think there ought to be some way to pay providers just a little bit better and have that network of providers for that population without standing up a clinic with walls. That is, there must be a network available in the community already that would be willing to see those patients and able to see those patients within existing facilities without having to stand up the walls of a clinic and pay a clinic administrator and all of the overhead associated with a clinic. Is any work being done in that area to sort of establish a federally qualified health center without walls?

Mr. SMITH. I will ask the administrator to help me out. I think part of——

Mr. BURGESS. Well, clearly, Chairman Barton, if I could just add to that, said this is a more cost-effective way of delivering care. If we are able to keep the patient in the doctor's office, whether it be a federally qualified health center or a private office, it is cheaper than going to the emergency room where you have the highest overhead on the planet. So you know, maybe I am just more making an observation rather than asking a question. It would seem to me that if you can capture physician networks within a community that needs a federally qualified health center but doesn't have one, and if you just pay a little bit better, you are going to be able to place those patients within private offices and, as Mr. Walden pointed out, possibly save a ton of money in the process. I just think back to my own days in private practice. No one ever expects to make money on a Medicaid patient, and in fact, I think we have been told that by the previous iteration of CMS that was HCFA, we just expect you to go broke a little more slowly. And I think that was sort of the business model where this was set up.

But please feel free to respond to that, and again, it may be more of an observation on my part than a question. It just seems like when we are looking for a better way to do things, this would be a better way.

Mr. SMITH. A couple things. I think you are pointing out that the solution is outside Medicaid in terms of getting more Americans insured. And certainly, the President has offered a number of proposals that expand insurance in the first place. Within the Medicaid program, treating people and giving them access to care in a clinic or an FQHC or in the doctor's office instead of in the emergency room is a goal certainly we all share. And I think that part of that is it is going to come in a variety of different approaches.

And as we have expanded coverage, there have also been folks that want to know if Medicaid is paying its share. I think Medicaid is paying its share for the Medicaid recipients in the reimbursement system that we presently have. As I stated, Medicaid accounts for 64 percent of total patient-related reimbursement to FQHCs.

So I think Medicaid is paying its share, and I think Congress has made sure that Medicaid is paying its share in the PPS system, the supplemental payments above the managed care rates, et cetera. But the real goal everybody has is to expand insurance so people are seeking care in the most appropriate setting instead of in emergency rooms.

Mr. BURGESS. Well, is there a subset of the population that really just needs help buying insurance rather than the full faith and credit of the Medicaid system behind them?

Mr. SMITH. Again, I think what the President is proposing is to be able to expand coverage through a variety of different ways, whether it is through the employers, giving tax credits to small businesses, forming purchasing pools, or tax credits to help people meet the cost of care. They could take a variety of approaches, and the President, in his budget, has increased the Federal commitment to health care spending.

Mr. BURGESS. Mr. Chairman, I have taken more time—I am sorry. Did you have something you wanted to add, Dr. Duke?

Ms. DUKE. I just could add that we do have some models where centers have entered into partnerships with private providers. In Salt Lake City, 600 private providers work with the county, the hospitals, the doctors, and the health centers to do what you are talking about in the sense that the services are expanded by private contributions from doctors who take uninsured patients and provide those services as part of their commitment to the community.

Mr. BURGESS. Thank you, Mr. Chairman. I have used more time than I intended. I will yield back.

Mr. WHITFIELD. The gentleman from Washington, Mr. Inslee.

Mr. INSLEE. Thank you.

I wonder if either or both of you could talk about the clinics' experience with the Medicare prescription drug bill. What percentage of folks are signed up for that? What are not? What experience have you had with the bill that was adopted a while back?

Mr. SMITH. In terms of enrollment, there are a number of people who will automatically be enrolled, people who are presently eligible for Medicaid will be automatically enrolled into a plan. I don't believe the MMA had a specific provision about the role of the FQHCs, but certainly at CMS and HRSA, we are encouraging PDPs and the plans to include FQHCs in their network. FQHCs in particular play a very vital role in access for individuals, and we are certainly encouraging that. For enrollment of the rest of the Medicare population, we are on the threshold of the Social Security Administration and CMS doing great outreach efforts to encourage individuals to apply for the low-income subsidy so that Medicare will pay the vast majority of the cost of enrolling in the part D prescription drugs. We are encouraging the plans to make the FQHCs a part of their network. So we don't have statistics yet on actual enrollment, because we are at the beginning of that for the entire population.

Mr. INSLEE. So can you give me any flavor at all? Are people rushing to sign up on their first visits to the health center, or is this a hard sell? Or can you give me any flavor of what is happening out there?

Ms. DUKE. I have just, within the last week, sent out a letter to health centers to initiate this process, so we are really at the very beginning, and I have no data on that at this point. But as we get data, I will be glad to share it with you.

Mr. INSLEE. Have you had any feedback from the health centers about the relative response to their constituents at all to this effort?

Ms. DUKE. No, I just sent the letter out within the last week.

Mr. SMITH. If I may add, I believe that with Social Security's capabilities, we are going to have very sophisticated analysis at the local level, by county, to be able to identify the take-up rates. As we have said, we are at the very beginning of that, but over time, those will be targeted. We have teams around the country who will continue to look at that data to make certain that the take-up rates are as positive as possible.

So if we see that enrollment is lagging behind, we have teams that will then provide outreach to sign up the beneficiaries.

Mr. INSLEE. So you haven't gotten calls from the health centers that they are overwhelmed and you have got to put on new help to get people clamoring to get on that? It doesn't sound like it anyway.

Mr. SMITH. We have a whole variety of different agencies involved in the outreach including Social Security and SHIPs. We have the area agencies on aging. The FQHCs are part of a very large effort to do the outreach.

Mr. INSLEE. Well, I suspect you won't be overwhelmed with the needs of people to process this, so that probably won't be a problem.

Thank you.

Mr. SMITH. Thank you.

Mr. WHITFIELD. Ms. Blackburn, you are recognized for 10 minutes.

Ms. BLACKBURN. Thank you, Mr. Chairman.

And I am going to try to consolidate this as much as I can, so that we get through everyone before we go to vote.

And Mr. Smith, you said something earlier that I think hits the nail on the head with the centers that I have seen, and that is that when you have the type of access that these centers provide then you do have a lower cost. I think the other thing that I have noticed in the centers is the environment. And you create an environment where there is an acceptance that it is okay to ask questions and to get some education on how to deal with health care situations. And I think that is a positive as we look for ways to better educate.

Mr. Smith, one more thing before I go to Dr. Duke.

The revenue stream, we have talked around that a couple of times, and you mentioned 36 percent of the funding comes from Medicaid payments, Medicare and Medicaid. If you will just in writing for me later, break that stream down as to how most centers arrive at their full funding.

And then I want to move on to my risk management liability questions that I have.

And Dr. Duke, the HHSIG's report from February 2005 talks about HSRA no longer performing onsite primary care effectiveness reviews and that HSRA is developing a new performance assessment protocol for all its grantees, including the health centers. And what I would like to know is if this has been developed and if it has not, when it is to be developed and fully implemented.

Ms. DUKE. We are in the process now of doing the first full year of performance reviews for our grantees. The approach we have taken is to do one review per grantee and to cover all of the grants that they might have from us so that perhaps they have a health center grant, they might have an HIV/AIDS grant, so that we would not go back twice to the same grantee. We would do them all at once.

Ms. BLACKBURN. So your new model will be one onsite review.

Ms. DUKE. Yes.

Ms. BLACKBURN. Then the balance, are you planning to handle that as a web-based review or information submission or what is your template?

Ms. DUKE. The approach we have taken is that the reviews actually use both.

Ms. BLACKBURN. Okay.

Ms. DUKE. That is to say there is a preparatory stage, which is document reviews, web-based, and so forth, and then there is an onsite, and then there is a feedback process, and it has been received very well by grantees as positive.

Ms. BLACKBURN. Okay. Great. I will be interested in following that. I think that is an important part of this concept as we look at the care delivery, the cost-effectiveness, and increasing the scope of the program.

In that vein, you have got 33 percent of the centers that have received accreditation from the Joint Commission of Health Care Organizations. Okay. And when do you think you are going to have all current centers or your grant recipients receiving accreditation?

Ms. DUKE. We are working very closely in trying to move that forward. We have a goal of having 100 percent coverage, but we won't reach it this year.

Ms. BLACKBURN. Are all of the centers actively pursuing accreditation or——

Ms. DUKE. I don't believe I could say all of them are seeking accreditation at this point. There are issues of cost involved.

Ms. BLACKBURN. Okay.

Ms. DUKE. And so I think at this point, people are balancing many competing demands, but that is our goal is that we will reach that. But we won't reach it this year.

Ms. BLACKBURN. Okay. Let us quickly talk about risk management controls, because the Inspector General's report notes that the risk management training is lacking. And I will ask you to respond to this in writing, because we are in the vote. I would like to know how the centers are conducting their risk management training workshops and if you all have a comprehensive agenda for covering that risk management.

And then my final question to you will be, and you can respond in writing to this, too, just for the interest of time, looking at the health center tort claims fund from which the malpractice claims are paid. And I would like to know the current status of that fund and what is the average amount of a malpractice claim on one of the centers?

And with that, Mr. Chairman, I will yield back.

Mr. WHITFIELD. Thank you.

Mr. STUPAK. Mr. Chairman, before we yield, you were asking questions on the OIG report. Do you have that, and could you put it in the record so we could have that?

Ms. BLACKBURN. Yes, I do have that, and I will be happy to put it in the record.

Mr. STUPAK. Okay. Thank you.

Mr. WHITFIELD. Without objection, so ordered.

Mr. Green, you are recognized.

Mr. GREEN. Thank you, Mr. Chairman, and I will try and be brief, because I know we have a vote in a little over 2 minutes.

One, I want to thank you and the ranking member for allowing me to be on the subcommittee. I serve on the Health Subcommittee, and obviously community health centers are important, and I want to thank HRSA for the ten for Texas and we received five in the Houston area. We have identified, through Dr. Sanchez, who used to be our Health Commissioner. I don't know what we call him now since the State legislature merged all of the agencies, identified community-based clinics as a way that we can deal with it with the resources that we don't have. But it brings it down to the local level oftentimes that, for example, the one that was just awarded in Pasadena had fund-raisers and we had both business and, in fact, one of our for-profit hospitals convinced that over half their emergency room contacts could be eliminated by having a community health clinic. And our numbers, we think 57 percent of the emergency room visits in Houston and Harris Counties are people who could have been served by a community-based clinic. And so I agree that we could look at lowering some of our other costs if we do that.

One of the concerns I have is we have been looking at, in the success we had, two of those five were in the District I represent. And what I was trying to see, is it easier for FQHCs to have amendments or look-alikes than it is to have another free-standing one, because it seems like maybe they would have better response from HRSA for expansion? So if we only have five, for example, in the city of Houston and we are looking at the next round to see what we can do, is it better to have just expansions of clinics, additional sites that are in the needy areas, or it seems like it is much harder to get a whole new free-standing clinic with a new board?

Ms. DUKE. The look-alikes often make very good candidates for actual grant status in the sense that they already meet many of the same requirements. And so I don't think that the question is mutually exclusive. I think moving to look-alike status has the advantage of providing care and getting some benefits from the Federal Government and then being able to compete very well. Look-alikes have competed very well for those grants.

Mr. GREEN. Okay. The other issue for the one of the clinics, I know the funding doesn't begin until later this year, and I know in 2005, Congress provided $775 billion for community health centers, and I know that several programs, the Bureau of Primary Health Care, have it delayed during the current fiscal year. And can you explain how the fiscal year 2005 funding for community health centers has been allocated or is being allocated? It looks like the 330 grants are being moved into the next budget year.

Ms. DUKE. We have the costs of continuing the grantees we already have, which is a number of about almost 3,700. And so they continue to get grants to continue their operations. And so the issue is the availability of funds to start new centers. One of the issues, for me, or at least my sense, is that there is a terrible cost for people that have to keep coming in to compete over and over again. And so one of the things we have tried to do was to identify the groups who had already competed successfully and to identify them for funding in the next round rather than go through another very costly grant process so that we, in essence, have one leg up on the next cycle.

Mr. GREEN. And Mr. Chairman, my last statement is if we use the cap program to put together these collaboratives for the community, and I know the President is supporting community-based clinics, but we also need the cap program to be able to put together these collaboratives, particularly in areas that we have to bring the community groups and the folks together on.

But Mr. Smith, my last question for CMS is two of the FQHCs in my District have expressed frustration with the process of obtaining Medicaid provider numbers for Federal reimbursement. There was a merger between two of our clinics, and it took 7 months to get a provider number. Is there some way that if you have two clinics, for example, that may have separate numbers that it could be fast-tracked on instead of the delay sometimes?

Mr. SMITH. Mr. Green, that is Medicare. Medicare is enrolling the providers directly. I would be happy to get back to you on that.

Mr. GREEN. Okay.

Mr. SMITH. I just don't know off hand.

Mr. GREEN. I know our own experiences with our one in Pasadena, we needed the number very quickly, and thank goodness there is a Texan who I know is family who runs CMS, and we were able to get that number quickly, but not everybody can call their Member of Congress and get it done.

Mr. SMITH. If you could give me their names, I will make sure we check them.

Mr. GREEN. Okay. We can get that information to you.

Mr. SMITH. Okay.

Mr. GREEN. In fact, when we run vote, my staff will be able to share it.

Mr. SMITH. We will be happy to follow up.

Mr. GREEN. And again, thank you, Mr. Chairman, for letting me in. It is a great——

Mr. WHITFIELD. Thank you, Mr. Green.

We do have a series of four votes on the floor. We had a lot of other questions for you, Dr. Duke, and Mr. Smith, but we are not going to ask you to stay, because we have another panel coming in. But we are going to submit some additional questions in writing, particularly for you, Mr. Smith, and one being, for example, should States be allowed to spend Medicaid dollars to establish community health centers themselves, meeting the guidelines? Just something to think about. And we will have some additional questions for you.

And then Dr. Duke, one thing that I would like to ask you all to provide us is 2003/2004 list of new grantees by Congressional District. If you would do that, we would appreciate it. And Mr. Stupak, do you have anything?

Mr. STUPAK. Not at this time.

Mr. WHITFIELD. Okay. Okay. And like I said, we will submit additional questions in writing.

And thank you all so much, and we look forward to continue working with you as we strive to improve health care.

And with that, the first panel is dismissed.

For those of you on the second panel, as I said, we have four votes. We are going to go cast those votes now. I imagine we could be back here by about 4:35. And we will swear you in at that point, and we will begin your panel.

So thank you very much.

With that, we are in recess.

[Brief recess.]

Mr. WHITFIELD. Okay. On our second panel, we have Mr. Roderick Manifold, who is the Executive Director at the Central Virginia Health Services, Incorporated; Mrs. Kim Sibilsky, who is the Executive Director of the Michigan Primary Care Association; Mr. Daniel Hawkins, who is the Vice-President of the National Association of Community Health Centers; Dr. Janelle Goetcheus, who is the Medical Director of Unity Health Care; and Dr. Leiyu Shi, who is an Associate Professor at Johns Hopkins School of Public Health. We welcome all of you.

And where is Mr. Manifold? Okay. Well, Mr. Stupak has just come back from voting as well, and so as soon as we get Mr. Manifold, we will go on and have you sworn in and you can begin your testimony.

And we do genuinely thank you for being with us today, and we look forward to hearing what you have to say.

I will tell you, if it is going to be 10 minutes, we will go on and swear these in, and we will go on and start with your testimony.

So I will call the meeting back to order. And you all are aware that this is an investigative hearing, and it is the practice of the Oversight Investigations Subcommittee that we give testimony under oath. Do any of you have any difficulty giving testimony under oath? And you also know that when you give it under oath, if you want legal counsel, you have that right. And assuming you do not have legal counsel, so if you will stand, I will swear you in.

[Witnesses sworn.]

Mr. WHITFIELD. Thank you. Okay. You are now under oath, and Mrs. Sibilsky, we will start with you. And be sure and turn your microphone on and get it up close. And you may begin your 5-minute opening statement.

TESTIMONY OF KIM SIBILSKY, EXECUTIVE DIRECTOR, MICHIGAN PRIMARY CARE ASSOCIATION; DANIEL R. HAWKINS, JR., VICE-PRESIDENT, NATIONAL ASSOCIATION OF COMMUNITY HEALTH CENTERS; A. JANELLE GOETCHEUS, MEDICAL DIRECTOR, UNITY HEALTH CARE; LEIYU SHI; AND RODERICK V. MANIFOLD, EXECUTIVE DIRECTOR, CENTRAL VIRGINIA HEALTH SERVICES, INC.

Ms. SIBILSKY. Good afternoon. My name is Kim Sibilsky, and I am the Executive Director of the Michigan Primary Care Association.

On behalf of Michigan's federally qualified health centers, I thank you for this opportunity to testify.

Representing community-based primary care centers, MPCA provides a myriad of services, including health professional recruitment, clinical support, technical assistance services, education and training, as well as assisting organizations becoming community migrant health centers or other primary care delivery models. In short, we are a membership association of FQHCs dedicated to educating for the medically under-served.

Mr. Chairman and members of the subcommittee, I believe the most important job of a health center is to serve as a medical home for medically under-served communities. In Michigan, health centers serve as the medical home and are delivering comprehensive primary care to more than 425,000 persons in more than 140 communities and neighborhoods. Our 29 FQHC organizations form an essential component of the State's safety net for health care services. To that end, we are committed to bringing high-quality, comprehensive health care to people and communities in Michigan that desperately need them.

This job is getting tougher every day, however. Growing health care costs coupled with increased uninsured and underinsured people in Michigan and nationwide directly contributes to the growing number of Medicaid-eligible people. In Michigan, nearly 25 percent of the State's low-income residents lack basic health insurance. And about 12 percent of the overall State population is uninsured.

Seen another way, unless these people are fortunate enough to live in a community with an FQHC or a free or a charity clinic, they have few options, other than their local hospital's emergency room, to receive care. And let me tell you, there are consequences to this reality.

In 2001, Michigan looked at preventable hospitalizations, those for which timely and effective ambulatory care can help reduce the risks for common problems, such as asthma, diabetes, or dehydration. High rates of preventable hospitalizations in a community signal potential barriers to care, including lack of sufficient primary care resources.

The review estimated that Michigan had over 240,000 preventable hospitalizations, which resulted in almost 1.3 million unnecessary inpatient days of care. But this does not have to be the reality today. FQHCs strategically placed in under-served communities increase access to early intervention and improve the economic and physical health of Michigan's communities.

Through the President's initiative, Michigan has expanded access to care to over 56,000 residents in 28 communities. As Michigan's uninsured population continues to grow, the State also is experiencing record levels of enrollment in Medicaid as the result of our slow economic recovery. Currently, Michigan's Medicaid program covers one out of seven citizens. With such high Medicaid enrollment numbers and low State revenues, the pressure is on to identify cost savings.

Mr. Chairman, FQHCs stand ready to be a part of the answer. In Michigan alone, 29 FQHC organizations currently care for 10 percent of all Medicaid enrollees for less than 1 percent of the physician services budget. In other words, health centers are saving the Medicaid program money.

This achievement is made possible largely because of Congress' wise decision to support adequate Medicaid reimbursement to health centers by creating the prospective payment system for FQHCs. I am proud to say that the implementation of the prospective payment system is a huge success, and we applaud Congress for their support.

However, as Congress considers to Medicaid, it is critical that it recognize the unique relationship between health centers and Medicaid. In particular, lawmakers must appreciate the changes in Medicaid that could be construed as minor could actually have devastating impacts on health centers. For example, the elimination of dental services for Medicaid adults in Michigan in 2003 is still causing tremendous stress to the system and to health centers. And to be sure, Michigan's Medicaid adult benefit waiver program continues to threaten FQHCs' abilities to protect Federal dollars for the uninsured in the State. Lawmakers must be careful not to inadvertently impact the mission of health centers during discussions on Medicaid reform.

And I, along with the Michigan health centers, look forward to working with Congress in this effort.

Thank you for this opportunity to talk with you. If there are any questions, I would be pleased to answer.

[The prepared statement of Kim E. Sibilsky follows:]

PREPARED STATEMENT OF KIM SIBILSKY, EXECUTIVE DIRECTOR, MICHIGAN PRIMARY CARE ASSOCIATION ON BEHALF OF THE MICHIGAN PRIMARY CARE ASSOCIATION

Good Afternoon. My name is Kim Sibilsky and I am here representing Michigan's Federally Qualified Health Centers (FQHC), which include community, migrant, homeless health centers. I am the Executive Director of the Michigan Primary Care Association (MPCA). The MPCA is a nonprofit organization developed to promote, support and develop comprehensive, accessible and affordable, quality primary health care services to everyone living in Michigan. Representing organizational providers and affiliates of community-based primary care centers in the state, we provide a myriad of services, including health professional recruitment, clinical support and technical assistance services, education and training as well as helping organizations become a Community/Migrant Health Center or other primary care delivery model.

Thank you for this opportunity to speak with you today.

Federally Qualified Health Centers (FQHC) provide medical homes to residents of medically underserved communities. Michigan's health centers deliver comprehensive primary care in more than 140 Michigan communities and neighborhoods to more than 425,000 persons. Michigan's 29 FQHC organizations form an essential component of the state's safety net for health care services. We are committed to providing high quality, comprehensive health care services to federally designated medically underserved areas and populations.

As FQHC organizations, we provide a comprehensive set of primary care services and enabling services to all people, regardless of their ability to pay. Our clinics not only provide care to families, they also provide care to high risk and special populations including people with changing insurance coverage and those with chronic conditions and disabilities. Research has repeatedly shown that these groups cost the system a disproportionate share of available resources and we are committed to providing them with the best service in a cost-effective manner.

To address the cost of health care, we must ensure that necessary services are available, are delivered by the most appropriate provider, and are accessible in the most cost-effective setting, at the right time. By regulation, only communities lacking such access qualify for a Federally Qualified Health Center. These regulations focus on two different, but equally important issues: 1) a severe shortage of primary care providers for the entire community; and/or 2) a severe shortage due to primary care physicians refusing to provide essential care to populations in need.

Research shows that you can reduce the cost of health care by increasing access to preventive and primary care services. It follows that a reduction in health care costs will result in a reduction in the number of uninsured persons. Yet the cost of health care continues to grow and the growing number of uninsured and underinsured people in Michigan and across the country is directly contributing to the growing number of Medicaid eligible people. This results in a burgeoning Medicaid budget. Figures calculated from the Current Population Survey and Claritas, a data clearinghouse, indicate that more than 250,000 or 24.7% of Michigan's low-income residents lack basic health insurance. Looking at all income levels, 1.1 million or 12% of Michigan's residents and 45 million or 15.6% nationally are uninsured.

Unless an uninsured person is fortunate enough to live in a community with an FQHC or a free/charity clinic, they have few options other than their local hospital's emergency room. Reports indicate that 58% percent of the 106,000,000 annual visits to hospital emergency rooms across the country are described as inappropriate. In a new study published in Health Services Research; entitled, "ailability of Safety Net Providers and Access to Care of Uninsured Persons" Hadley J. and Cunningham P., October 2004) finds that FQHCs are more cost effective because they improve access to primary care for the uninsured and underinsured and reduce emergency room visits and hospital stays.

Michigan completed a study in 2001 which looked at preventable hospitalizations, those for which timely and effective ambulatory care can help reduce the risks for common problems such as asthma, diabetes or dehydration. High rates of preventable hospitalizations in a community signal potential barriers to care including lack of sufficient primary care resources. The review estimated that we had over 240,000 preventable hospitalizations which resulted in almost 1.3 million unnecessary inpatient days of care.

Michigan's Medicaid program covers 1 out of 7 citizens. We continue to experience record levels of enrollment as a result of our slow economic recovery. With such high Medicaid enrollment numbers and low state revenues, the pressure is on to identify cost savings. FQHCs stand ready to be a part of the answer. Several studies have demonstrated that health centers save the Medicaid program more than 30% in annual spending per beneficiary due to reduced specialty care referral and fewer hospital admissions and FQHCs save by helping to prevent unnecessary usage of the emergency room. Studies have indicated that Medicaid beneficiaries who sought care at health centers were 22% less likely to be hospitalized for potentially avoidable conditions than beneficiaries who obtained care elsewhere. *Michigan's 29 FQHC organizations currently care for 10% of all Medicaid enrollees for less than 1% of the physician services budget.*

Federally Qualified Health Centers (FQHC) applaud the work of Congress to protect the federal funds provided to help care for the uninsured and underinsured. From the beginning, Congress recognized that without mandating a payment system that provided sufficient resources to the FQHCs to care for Medicaid clients, federal dollars may be shifted away from the uninsured. Previously, this meant cost-based reimbursement. On January 1, 2001, the Prospective Payment System outlined in the Medicare and Medicaid Beneficiaries Improvement and Protection Act of 2000 was implemented across the country. This was a historic moment in our program's history. For Michigan FQHCs, not only did this allow them to plan for the future with a predictable budget, it created incentives to innovate and implement cost-saving programs such as the 340(b) drug pricing program. FQHCs welcomed and continue to support efforts to maximize the use of limited tax dollars at both the state and federal levels. The Prospective Payment System is key to these efforts.

Under the Prospective Payment System, each FQHC is assigned a prospective payment amount calculated from their reported 1999-2000 costs. While states have implemented the system in slightly different ways, they all are required to adjust the rates annually by at least the Medicare Economic Index (MEI). These adjustments have averaged around 2.7% over the last four years, way below the medical inflation rate. Even with these modest adjustments, Michigan FQHCs view the implementation of the Prospective Payment System as a huge success and support efforts by our State Medicaid Agency to act as a guardian on behalf of the public good. We have to work within a budget and we understand that both the State and federal government have to do the same.

The Prospective Payment System reimburses the FQHCs and FQHC "look-alikes" on an encounter basis. FQHC encounters combine the cost of the face-to-face visit with a provider and the cost of ancillary services such as immunizations, on-site lab and x-rays, translation, and nutritional counseling provided during the visit into one payment. People not directly involved in the FQHC program often mistakenly believe that we are paid higher rates for office visits than private physician offices. In reality, private physician offices usually do not provide the scope of services we do and when they do provide some of these ancillary services, they often do not incorporate these services into their practice without a means to receive payment.

Michigan would like to draw your attention to how crucial the Prospective Payment System is to FQHCs. We recognize that through the waiver process, states regularly request the ability to waive their obligation to provide FQHCs with payment according to the Prospective Payment System. This waiver activity has the potential to jeopardize the entire system. For example, when the State Children's Health Insurance Program was created, recognition of our payment system was not included. At the time of development, we anticipated that the enrollees would be relatively inexpensive to care for given that they were children. To our surprise, Michigan created a SCHIP waiver program for childless adults with incomes below 35% of the federal poverty level. This program is referred to as the Adult Benefits Waiver. As you can imagine, this is a very different population than the one we, and we believe Congress, envisioned. Adults enrolled in this program often have multiple conditions including chronic illness, substance abuse, and mental health issues. Many of them are very transient, moving from shelter to shelter or reside on the street. Without recognition of our Prospective Payment System, programs such as Michigan's Adult Benefit Waiver threaten the FQHCs' ability to protect the federal dollars for the uninsured persons in our communities. Because of the demographics of the target population, most private providers do not wish to enroll in these provider networks. As a result, more than half to two-thirds of the Adult Benefit Waiver program enrollees are patients of FQHCs. Recognition of our payment system would protect the financial viability of our nation's health centers and the federal funds provided for the uninsured.

I would like to ask for your assistance as you and your colleagues begin to evaluate the Medicaid program to remember the Federally Qualified Health Centers. Changes that could be construed as minor could have devastating impacts on our system. For example, the State of Michigan elected to eliminate dental services for Medicaid adults on October 1, 2003. This saved relatively little general fund dollars ($9.2 million) and would impact few providers given the relatively small number of private dentists enrolled in the program. What they did not understand is that the Federally Qualified Health Centers accounted for the majority of dental care currently being provided to the Medicaid adults. The elimination of Medicaid adult dental is still causing tremendous stress to our system since the need did not disappear, just the payment.

Everyone is struggling with how to pay for our Medicaid system. We must remember the interplay between publicly-funded coverage and the uninsured. When you restrict enrollment in public programs, the cost of providing care does not disappear and the savings are not absolute. People will eventually receive the care they need. It may not be in the best and most cost-effective location, at a time when the progression of illness can be headed off and the most expensive care prevented, but in the end, anyone can walk into a community hospital and receive some level of care. Our goal as providers is to squeeze any waste out of the system that we can. We believe a sizeable amount of waste exists simply from the vast amount of paperwork required of health care providers, the lack of connections between different components of the health care delivery system, and the mobility of our population. I would like to talk to you today about two opportunities that Michigan's FQHCs have embraced to help us address some of these challenges—the chronic disease collaboratives and technology.

Federally Qualified Health Centers are uniquely positioned to embrace change. Our administrators are particularly adept at stretching dollars, our clinicians are mission-oriented and employed by the centers, our Boards of Directors are made of a majority of users of the clinics and therefore personally committed to their continuation, and the federal government is an important partner with resources that go beyond the financial. With the support of the Bureau of Primary Health Care, the FQHCs have undertaken a major shift in how chronically ill patients are cared for and given the responsibility for their own health. Many positive changes have occurred as a result of the Chronic Disease Collaboratives. Some of these are listed below:

- Michigan Health Centers in the Chronic Disease Collaboratives have experienced drastic reductions in the severity of diabetes among their patients. The Hemoglobin A1c, a lab measurement used to gauge the severity of diabetes, has increased by 26% from the when the centers began to implement the model in 1999 to April 2005.
- Presently there are over 5,463 Michigan patients being tracked related to cardiovascular disease. The Chronic Disease Collaborative aims to reduce blood pressure which leads to reduction in complications associated with cardiovascular disease. To date, despite an influx in the number of new patients enrolled, the program has demonstrated a 5% overall increase in the number of patients with a blood pressure less than 140/90.
- In addition to tracking diabetes and cardiovascular disease, the Michigan health centers are spreading the care model to other chronic diseases including cancer, depression, asthma and a perinatal pilot project.

As a State Primary Care Association, we are working to educate our state policymakers about this program and in fact have a proposal pending with the State of Michigan that will draw many different provider types into providing care using the chronic care model including Critical Access Hospitals, community hospitals, independent and provider-based Rural Health Clinics, private physician offices, Medicaid Health Maintenance Organizations, and community-based coverage programs. This model has tremendous potential that is just beginning to be broadly appreciated such as improvements in patients' depressive symptoms, percentage increases of patients receiving appropriate treatment for chronic conditions and the ability to track measurable improvement in meeting nationally accepted guidelines. We are committed to providing assistance and sharing our lessons learned in order to see the impressive results in improvement of health status and reduction of health disparities in Michigan that we have experienced in health centers nationally.

Finally, in light of the national interest in moving health care to the electronic age, I'd like to speak with you concerning Michigan health centers' innovation in information technology supported by the Bureau of Primary Health Care of HRSA, VirtualCHC. VirtualCHC is an Application Service Provider (ASP) designed by MPCA which delivers application functionality and computer services to many users via the Internet or a private network. VirtualCHC houses software appropriate to health centers, including a number of choices of practice management, general ledger, Microsoft Office Suite and many others, making them available to health centers via the Internet.

As I mentioned earlier, electronic health records represent an opportunity. They are key to our efforts to improve the quality of care through better and more regular monitoring of patient/provider adherence to clinical guidelines and to eliminate duplication of services/testing/treatment. Implementing electronic health records is a large front-end expense for centers purchasing the software, equipment, training and lost productivity. VirtualCHC provides a way to help minimize that initial investment by giving them a viable alternative to developing and implementing complex systems themselves. Finally, because VirtualCHC is Internet based, there are no geographic limitations in health centers selecting or being supported by VirtualCHC. As a result, VirtualCHC has serviced health center clients in Michigan, Missouri, Massachusetts, Alaska and the Virgin Islands. With Community Health Centers, the future really IS now.

Thank you for this opportunity to talk with you. If there are any questions, I would be pleased to answer them at this time.

Mr. WHITFIELD. Thank you.

Mr. Hawkins, you are recognized for 5 minutes.

TESTIMONY OF DANIEL R. HAWKINS, JR.

Mr. HAWKINS. Thank you, Mr. Chairman.

Good afternoon to you and members of the subcommittee. My name is Dan Hawkins, and on behalf of America's health centers and their 15 million patients, thank you for the opportunity to speak with you this afternoon about the Federal health centers program and to share their success stories.

Mr. Chairman, I have personally seen the power of health centers to transform the health and well being of under-served people and communities as a VISTA volunteer back in the 1960's. I helped a community in a small, rural south Texas town to startup a health center and then served as its initial Director. That center is still in operation today, no thanks to me. It serves more than 40,000 people a year.

Conceived in 1965 as a bold experiment to bring health care services to our Nation's neediest communities, the health center program has a 40-year record of success, providing an enduring model of primary care delivery for the country.

Health centers have used community empowerment, what we like to call patient democracies, to produce improved health outcomes and quality of life. Dr. Duke has already pointed out the stellar record of achievement of the health centers. NAC, and all health centers, are deeply grateful to Congress for its support of the health centers program and for expanding its reach. The $566 million increase in appropriations provided since fiscal year 2002 has enabled more than 700 communities to secure a new or expanded health center, adding 4 million new patients over the last 4 years.

Program funds are rewarded nationally on a competitive basis, thus ensuring high-quality projects. Thankfully, Congress has also provided additional funding for existing centers, all of which face growing uninsured patient rolls and rising costs. We appreciate the President's historic request, a $304 million increase for next year. It can't come soon enough, as the numbers show. As you have heard earlier today, last year, over 430 applications were submitted for a new health center site, and only 91 of them received funding.

We are delighted the President has announced a second health center initiative to place a new health center in every poor county that currently lacks one. We recently released a study showing 929 such counties, including 69 in Kentucky and 11 in Michigan, several in your District, Mr. Chairman, and several in Mr. Stupak's District.

We look forward to working with the President and Congress to help this program reach every community in need. As my colleague, Kim Sibilsky has already noted, NAC and State primary care associations have long recognized that the success of the program and the current expansion initiatives will depend on the ability of health centers to meet all requirements and performance standards and expectations. With this in mind, we have significantly enhanced our training and technical assistance activities for health centers focused on financial management, clinical practice, and board governance, among others. We continue to assist hundreds of communities to successfully apply for new health center funding.

As you know, the health centers program is scheduled for reauthorization next year. Over the years, Congress has consistently reaffirmed and strengthened the core elements of the health centers program, including community governance, location in underserved communities, open-door policy regardless of health status, insurance coverage, or ability to pay, and focus on community-wide health. We believe these core statutory requirements provide the crucial framework for the success of the program. It simply would not be where it is today without them, and we commend the committee for consistently safeguarding these requirements over the years.

I want to turn, for a moment, to the Medicaid program. Medicaid health centers have long enjoyed a special relationship as twin pillars of a broad strategy to improve health care for the poor, minority, and under-served Americans. Today, that unique relationship continues with health centers caring for nearly 6 million Medicaid recipients, more than one of every ten Medicaid beneficiaries for less than 1 percent of all Medicaid dollars, while Medicaid serves as their single largest revenue source. Recognizing the importance of this relationship, Congress, in 1989, made health center services a guaranteed Medicaid benefit and required that its payments cover the cost of care for Medicaid patients so that their Federal grant funds could be dedicated to care of the uninsured. Since that time, health centers have doubled the number of uninsured people served to 6 million because Medicaid paid its fair share. And in 2000, this committee led Congress to reaffirm the importance of adequate Medicaid payments to health centers by creating a prospective payment system for them.

Today, health centers continue to deliver significant savings to all payers, and especially to Medicaid. They control health care costs by providing primary care and preventive services, reducing the need for more costly hospital care down the road. Dozens of studies have found that health centers save the Medicaid program 30 percent or more in total spending compared to other providers.

As Congress considers Medicaid reforms, we stand ready to work with the committee to ensure that any such reforms preserves Medicaid's crucial coverage for those who need it most and recognizes the key role of health centers in both caring for Medicaid recipients and the uninsured.

Thank you, once again, for this opportunity, and I would be happy to answer any questions.

[The prepared statement of Daniel R. Hawkins, Jr. follows:]

PREPARED STATEMENT OF DANIEL R. HAWKINS, JR., VICE PRESIDENT, FEDERAL, STATE, AND PUBLIC AFFAIRS, NATIONAL ASSOCIATION OF COMMUNITY HEALTH CENTERS

Mr. Chairman and Members of the Subcommittee, my name is Dan Hawkins and I am Vice President for Federal, State, and Public Affairs for the National Association of Community Health Centers. On behalf of America's Health Centers and the 15 million patients they serve, I want to express my gratitude for the opportunity to speak to you today about the federal Health Centers program. NACHC and health centers appreciate the unwavering support that this Subcommittee and the entire Committee has given to carry out their mission and we look forward to continuing to work with you to further strengthen the program to serve medically underserved communities. As the Committee that oversees not just the authorization of the Health Centers program, but also the entire Medicaid program, we appreciate the opportunity to appear before you today.

Mr. Chairman, I have personally seen the power of health centers to lift the health and the lives of individuals and families in our most underserved communities. As a VISTA volunteer assigned to south Texas in the 1960s, the residents of our town asked me to work on improving access to health care and clean water in our community. We decided to apply for funds through a relatively new, innovative program—the Migrant Health program. I stayed on and served as executive director of the health center from 1971 to 1977. The health center is still in operation today, and has expanded to serve over 40,000 patients annually. The community empowerment and patient-directed care model thrives today in every health center in America and I am honored to be here to share with you their success story.

Background and History of the Health Centers Program

Conceived in 1965 as a bold, new experiment in the delivery of health care services to our nation's most vulnerable populations, the Health Centers program has a 40-year record of success that serves as an endearing model of primary care delivery for the country. The Health Centers program began in rural Mississippi, and in inner-city Boston in the mid-1960s, to serve rural, migrant, and urban individuals who had little access to health care and no voice in the delivery of health services. In the 1980s and 1990s, the Health Care for the Homeless and Public Housing health centers were created. In 1996, the Community, Migrant, Public Housing and Health Care for the Homeless programs were consolidated into a single statutory authority within the Public Health Service Act (PHSA).

Congress established the program as a unique public-private partnership, and has continued to provide direct funding to community organizations for the development and operation of health systems that address pressing local health needs and meet national performance standards. This federal commitment has had a lasting and profound affect on health centers and the communities and patients they serve in every corner of the country. Now, as in 1965, health centers are designed to empower communities to create locally-tailored solutions that improve access to care and the health of the patients they serve.

This blueprint has stood the test of time, and has allowed health centers to serve hundreds of millions of people since the inception of the program. Health centers proudly accept this responsibility in return for the investment made by the American taxpayers in the form of PHSA grants. However, this overwhelmingly poor, uninsured, and medically underserved patient mix creates unique challenges for health centers that are not necessarily confronted by other health care providers.

Current Statistics

Indeed, America's Health Centers serve an estimated 15 million people in every state and territory. Health centers provide care to 10 million people of color, 6 million uninsured individuals, 700,000 seasonal and migrant farmworkers, and 600,000 homeless individuals. Over 1,000 health centers are located in 3,600 rural, frontier, and urban communities across the country. The communities served by health centers are in dire need of improved access to care, and in many cases the centers serve as the sole provider of health services in the area, including medical, dental, mental health, and substance abuse services.

Patients can walk through the doors of their local health center and receive one-stop health care delivery that offers a broad range of preventive and primary care services, including prenatal and well-child care, immunizations, disease screenings, treatment for chronic diseases such as diabetes, asthma, and hypertension, HIV testing, counseling and treatment, and access to mental health and substance abuse treatment. Health centers also offer critically important enabling services that ensure that health center patients can truly access care, such as family and community outreach, case management, translation and interpretation, and transportation services.

Delivery of High-Quality, Cost-Effective Care

Because of the unique model of patient empowerment, what we like to call "patient democracies", health centers have produced improved health outcomes and quality of life. Health centers provide preventive services to vulnerable populations that may not otherwise have access to certain services such as immunizations, health education, mammograms, and Pap smears, as well as colorectal, glaucoma, and other screenings. Health centers have also made significant headway in preventing anemia and lead poisoning.

Additionally, health centers have distinguished themselves in the management of chronic illness, meeting or exceeding nationally accepted practice standards for treatment of these conditions. In fact, the Institute of Medicine and the General Accounting Office have recognized health centers as models for screening, diagnosing, and managing chronic conditions such as cardiovascular disease, diabetes, asthma, depression, cancer, and HIV/AIDS.

HHS' Health Resources and Services Administration (HRSA) has also helped improve the provision of quality care at health centers through the Health Disparities Collaboratives initiative. At the end of 2004, more than two-thirds of all health centers had initiated this effort, and an additional 150 health centers have started a Collaborative this year. I like to think of the Collaboratives as clinical demonstrations for health centers, designed to improve the skills of clinical staff, and strengthen caregiving through the development of extensive patient registries that improve clinicians' ability to monitor the health of individual patients, and effectively educate patients on the self-management of their conditions. More than 75,000 people with chronic diseases have been enrolled in elective registries for cancer, diabetes, asthma, and cardiovascular disease. Health centers participating in the Collaboratives almost unanimously report that health outcomes for their patients have dramatically improved.

As a result of health centers' focus on the provision of preventive and primary care services and management of chronic diseases, low-income, uninsured health center users are more likely to have a usual source of care than the uninsured nationally. 99% of surveyed health center patients report that they were satisfied with the care they receive at health centers. Communities served by health centers have infant mortality rates between 10 and 40% lower than communities not served by health centers, and the latest studies have shown a continued decrease in infant mortality at health centers while the nationwide rate has increased. Health centers are also linked to improvements in accessing early prenatal care and reductions in low birth weight.

This one-stop, patient-centered approach works. The Health Centers program has been recognized by the Office of Management and Budget as one of the most effective and efficiently run programs in the Department of Health and Human Services (HHS). Numerous studies have also pointed to the success of health centers in reducing health disparities and improving the health status of vulnerable populations who receive care at their sites. Indeed, a major report by the George Washington University found that high levels of health center penetration among low-income populations generally results in the narrowing or elimination of health disparities in communities of color.

Historic Expansion of Access Through the Health Centers program

While health centers have had four decades of success, there has been no brighter moment in the life of the program than now. NACHC and health centers are deeply grateful to Congress for its support of the Health Centers program. In Fiscal Year (FY) 2005, Congress appropriated $1.7 billion in overall funding for the Health Centers program, a $566 million increase in funding over FY 2002.

These increases have enabled hundreds of additional communities to participate in the Health Centers program and to deliver community-based care to more than 4 million people in the past 4 years. We are also very grateful that Congress has provided additional funding for base grant adjustments for existing health centers, which have seen unexpected increases in the number of uninsured patients coming through their doors at the very same time they continue to battle the continuously rising cost of delivering health care in their communities. These base grant adjustments have allowed health centers across the country to stabilize their operations and continue to provide care to their existing patients, while also looking for ways to expand access to necessary care.

We also appreciate the President's strong support for the program and his historic request for a $304 million increase in FY 2006, which would bring overall health center funding to $2 billion. This year we expect health centers to serve nearly 16 million people in every state across the country. This would be a tremendous boost for those lacking care in their communities and we wholeheartedly support the Administration's request, which would meet the 5-year goal of the President to serve an additional 6.1 million patients at 1,200 new health centers.

Despite the expansion of the program, the demand for health centers is at record highs—in 2004, we estimate that there were over 430 applications for new access points, only 91 of which received funding—a 21 percent success rate, making health centers' funding on the same level with other competitively awarded grant programs under HHS. Indeed the application process is rigorous, and it should be. Health center program funds are awarded on a nationally competitive basis, ensuring that the highest possible quality projects receive approval. Organizations can apply for new access point funding (which is for new starts and new sites), or for expanded medical capacity funding to serve additional patients at existing sites, or to make new services such as dental or mental health services available to patients.

Given the increasing need for health centers, we are extremely grateful that the President has committed to continue the growth of program by announcing a continuation of his Health Center Initiative into the future. This new announcement will focus on placing new health centers in poor counties that currently lack a health center site, a very ambitious goal. To begin this effort, the President has requested $26 million in FY 2006 to fund 40 new access points in high need counties.

Given the President's new initiative, we have also examined the need in poor counties. NACHC and the George Washington University estimate that there are approximately 929 poor counties in need of a health center, from Kentucky to Michigan. Through this continued expansion, we believe that millions of additional patients would have access to care at a health centers. We commend the President for his continued support of the Health Centers program and we look forward to working with Congress to ensure it reaches every community in need.

Authorization of the Health Centers program

As we look forward in the life of this 40-year experiment in community health empowerment, I note that the Health Centers program was last reauthorized in 2002, as a part of the Health Care Safety Net Amendments Act. The program is scheduled for reauthorization next year. Health centers are grateful to the Committee for its leadership role in strengthening and improving the Section 330 statute in 2002, further modernizing it to serve millions of new patients. Most importantly, in reauthorizing the program the Committee and Congress reaffirmed its four core elements, as it has consistently over the entire life of the program. These core elements, which have greatly contributed to its continued success, require that health centers: 1) be governed by community boards a majority of whose members are current health center patients, to assure responsiveness to local needs; 2) be open to everyone in the communities they serve, regardless of health status, insurance coverage, or ability to pay; 3) be located in high-need medically-underserved areas; and 4) provide comprehensive preventive and primary health care services.

In reauthorizing these bedrock requirements, Congress sent a clear message that it sees patient involvement in health care service delivery as key to health centers' success in providing access and knocking down barriers to health care. Active patient management of health centers assures responsiveness to local needs. This begins with community empowerment, through the patient-majority governing board that manages health center operations and makes decisions on services provided, and leads to the fulfillment of the other core elements of the program.

Through the direction and input of these community boards, health centers can identify their communities' most pressing health concerns and work with their patients, providers, and other key stakeholders to address these issues. This has been particularly valuable as health centers address and work to eliminate health disparities in their patient population. Board members with unique and direct community connections determine the best approach for removing barriers to health care, helping health centers to meet their patients where they are, not where they want them to be. The critical, distinguishing feature of the health center model of community empowerment is that the community has been directly involved in virtually every aspect of the centers' operations, and, in turn, each health center has become an integral part of its community, identifying the most pressing community needs and either developing or advocating for the most effective business or public policy solutions.

I also want to expand on the other core features of the Section 330 program, each of which has played a key role in the continued success of the Health Centers program. First, health centers are unique among health providers and systems in its statutory requirement that they be open to all in the community regardless of ability to pay. Like the community board requirement, this element is what links health centers the local neighborhoods they serve. There is no cherry picking at health centers; everyone—the uninsured, underinsured, those on Medicaid and Medicare, and those who have private coverage can receive quality health care at health centers. Consequently, health centers have a very diverse payor mix, in which the federal grant constitutes approximately 25% of center revenues. Medicaid and SCHIP make up 40% of revenue, private insurance constitutes 15%, and Medicare approximately 6%. Health centers are interested in addressing health needs on a truly community-wide basis, and the requirement that they be open to all in the areas they serve allows them to do just that.

Second, health centers are required under the statute to be located in high-need, medically-underserved areas. In reauthorizing the provision in 2002, Congress sought to ensure that much-needed, precious resources are allocated to the communities most in need of the services of a health center. Location of health centers in MUAs prevents the duplication of services, and establishes health centers in newly identified communities or expands the work of existing centers where there are well-documented gaps in care.

Third, health centers are distinctive in the broad range of required and optional primary and preventive health and related services they provide under Section 330. This also includes a range of enabling services that ensure optimal access to care. In 2002, Congress not only reauthorized this requirement, but added to the list by including appropriate cancer screenings and specialty referrals as required services and behavioral health, mental health, substance abuse, and recuperative care treatment as optional services that health centers may provide.

We believe that these core statutory requirements provide the crucial framework for success of the Health Centers program. The program simply would not be where it is today without these critical elements, and we commend Congress for safeguarding these requirements in every reauthorization of the Section 330 since its inception.

Need for Construction Assistance

While health centers greatly appreciate the ongoing effort of the federal government to expand the reach of the program, we must acknowledge the growing need for support for facility construction, renovation, and modernization. Currently, we estimate that over two-thirds of health centers need to upgrade, expand, or replace their facilities. Approximately 30% of health center buildings are more than 30 years old and 65% operate in facilities that are more than 10 years old. The average cost of a facility project is estimated to be $1.8 million, but projects can range in size from a small $400,000 project to a major $20 million effort. NACHC estimates that the current unmet need among health centers for capital projects is approximately $1.2 billion.

We strongly believe that the delivery of quality care to patients at health centers hinges greatly upon the quality of the facilities where care is provided. Prior to 1996, health centers could use a small portion of their grant funding for construction, renovation, and modernization of their facilities; elimination of this authority during the 1996 reauthorization and the failure to restore it during the 2002 process has severely undermined health centers' ability to successfully address their most pressing capital needs. As just one example, wiring a health center for high-speed IT systems or secure wireless networks, which will be crucial as we move to electronic health records, is not an allowable grant cost today.

Given this limited access to capital resources, health centers were very pleased that the Bureau of Primary Care Loan Guarantee Program was revised as part of the 2002 reauthorization to allow health centers to use loans not only for the development of managed care networks, but also for the purchase of equipment and to refinance existing loans previously made for facility construction. However, these funds still cannot be used for capital projects, and the guarantee covers only 80% of the value of the loan. Consequently, health centers participation has been limited, as many centers find it difficult to cover 20% of initial loan value, because of very slim financial margins as non-profit organizations serving low-income, underserved populations.

Despite this, health centers have worked hard to leverage resources to participate in other federal programs that offer capital assistance. Health centers in rural areas have been very successful in obtaining funding for facility improvement from the Department of Agriculture's Rural Housing Administration programs, which provide loan guarantees up to 90% of loan value. Health centers have had more limited success in accessing facility assistance through the Department of Housing and Urban Development (HUD) programs. If health centers were able to access HUD's loan guarantee and mortgage insurance, they would have an important tool with which to address facility concerns. We look forward to working with Congress to ensure that health centers are given the tools to expand, modernize and, when needed, to build new facilities in order to serve additional patients.

Above all, we stand ready to assist the Committee as you move forward next year to reauthorize the Section 330 Health Centers program and its core elements.

The Importance of Health Centers and Medicaid

I want to turn for a moment to the importance of Medicaid to the Health Centers program. Since their creation back in 1965, Medicaid and health centers have enjoyed a special relationship, as twin pillars of a broad strategy whose goal was to dramatically improve health care for poor, minority, and underserved Americans. Today, that unique relationship continues: just as health centers rely on Medicaid revenues, Medicaid beneficiaries rely on health centers for their care. Health centers are major providers of primary and preventive care services in Medicaid today, caring for nearly six million Medicaid recipients. In fact, Medicaid is currently the single largest beneficiary of health center services, as well as health centers' single largest source of financing. Keenly recognizing the importance of health center services to Medicaid beneficiaries, Congress in the Omnibus Budget Reconciliation Act of 1989 made the services of a Federally Qualified Health Centers (FQHCs) a guaranteed Medicaid benefit offered to beneficiaries in every State Medicaid program. Most important, Congress recognized and acknowledged that Medicaid reimbursement to FQHCs must be sufficient to assure that health centers were paid their full reasonable costs for serving Medicaid patients (so that they would not have to use their Public Health Service Act grant funds to subsidize low Medicaid payments). In the accompanying Committee report, lawmakers wrote:

"The Subcommittee on Health and the Environment heard testimony that, on average, Medicaid payments to Federally-qualified health centers cover less than 70 percent of the costs incurred by the centers in serving Medicaid patients. The role of the programs funded under sections 329, 330, and 340 of the PHS Act is to deliver comprehensive primary care services to underserved populations or areas without regard to ability to pay. To the extent that the Medicaid program is not covering the cost of treating its own beneficiaries, it is compromising the ability of the centers to meet the primary care needs of those without any public or private coverage whatsoever." (U.S. Congress, 1989, p. 415).

In the 16 years since enactment of the FQHC Medicaid requirement, health centers have increased their capacity for uninsured care by 3 million people—double the number of uninsured patients served in 1990, a rate of growth that is more than twice that for the nation's uninsured population. Alternatively stated, the Congress has received a higher rate of return on its annual appropriations investment in health centers because Medicaid cost-based reimbursement was in place.

In 2000, under the leadership of former Republican Congressman (now Senator) Richard Burr and his Democratic colleague Congressman Edolphus Towns, and with the support of the overwhelming majority of the Energy and Commerce Committee, Congress reaffirmed the continued importance of adequate Medicaid reimbursement to health centers by creating a prospective payment system for FQHCs that (1) assures continued access to care for Medicaid patients, (2) protects Federal grant funds to provide care for the uninsured, and (3) gives state Medicaid agencies greater flexibility in designing their Medicaid programs and predictability in the cost of payments to health centers.

Today, health centers continue to deliver significant savings to all payers, and especially to Medicaid. They control health care costs by providing primary and preventive services, reducing the need for more costly hospital care down the road. In South Carolina, for example, the state health department analyzed their annual costs for patients who have diabetes as a primary or secondary diagnosis. They found that patients of CareSouth, a health center system that had participated in the Diabetes Collaborative, had annual health costs of $343.00 per patient, while patients of other providers had a cost of $1,600 and specialists had a cost of $1,900. The health center had produced those results by reducing the average blood sugar level of their diabetic patients from 11 to 8—a 3 point drop (a 1 point decrease translates into a 17% decrease in mortality, an 18% decrease in heart attacks, and a 15% decrease in strokes) (Health Resources and Services Administration, 2003).

In addition, according to another study, communities served by health centers had 5.8 *fewer preventable hospitalizations* per 1,000 people over three years than other medically underserved communities not served by a health center (Epstein, 2001). Another study found that Medicaid beneficiaries who seek care at health centers were 22 percent less likely to be hospitalized for potentially avoidable conditions than beneficiaries who obtained care elsewhere (Falik, 2001) Several other studies have found that health centers save the Medicaid program more than 30 percent in annual spending per beneficiary by successfully managing their patients' care in ways that reduce the need for, and use of, specialty care referrals and hospital admissions (Braddock, 1994: Duggar, 1994a; Duggar, 1994b; Falik, 2001; Starfield, 1994; Stuart, 1995; Stuart, 1993).

Growing Challenges

Beyond paying its fair share for health center services provided to beneficiaries, Medicaid plays an important role by providing its beneficiaries access to comprehensive services beyond those available at health centers. However, as the health care needs of low-income individuals continue to grow, so do the challenges to health centers in sustaining their ability to provide quality care to Medicaid beneficiaries and other patients.

Undoubtedly, one of the greatest of these challenges is the increasing number of states in the past few years that have sought to limit the scope and the breadth of services provided to enrollees in their state Medicaid programs as well as implementing so-called "cost-containment" measures. Cutbacks in Medicaid eligibility levels or benefits, caps in enrollment, or forgone expansion plans naturally are presenting significant difficulties for health centers. What's more, these actions are occurring at the same time as employers are either shifting more of the rising cost of health insurance onto their workers or to dropping the coverage altogether. As other health care providers have begun cutting back on the uncompensated or charity care they provide, the result is that health centers are serving an ever-increasing number of uninsured individuals who previously were covered under Medicaid or through their employers.

Compounding this challenge is the increasing level of discretion being provided to the states in the operation of their Medicaid programs through HHS' issuance of Section 1115 waivers—under which State Medicaid agencies are permitted to reduce benefits, increase cost sharing requirements, and adjust reimbursement rates. Health centers have already experienced the impact of this increased state flexibility in some fifteen states during the 1990s. In most cases, the ability of health centers to care for both their Medicaid and their uninsured patients during this period was negatively impacted when their Medicaid payments were reduced below the cost of providing care. In many of those states, other providers decided not to participate or limited their care to only a few Medicaid patients, leaving health centers as one of the few remaining sources of primary and preventive care to this population.

While these and other changes in the health care system have put a tremendous strain on the overall Health Centers program, health centers remained committed to providing access to care for everyone that walks through their doors, regardless of their health status, insurance coverage, or ability to pay for services. Put simply, health centers will continue to provide care for those whom other providers cannot or will not serve.

Health Centers and Medicaid Reform

As Congress moves forward on considering ways in which to reform Medicaid, it is critical that it keep in mind the important role health centers play in their communities and the unique relationship between these centers and the Medicaid program. Indeed, as the Kaiser Family Foundation points out, "[t]he fundamental interrelationship between Medicaid and health centers . . . suggests, by extension, that dynamics in one domain are bound to have important impacts in the other." It is therefore imperative that lawmakers working on Medicaid reform consider the impact of any changes in that program on the ability of health centers to fulfill their public policy mission.

All health care providers must seek to cross-subsidize when payments from a third party source are insufficient. However, unlike most physician practices that have paid for indigent care services by cross-subsidies from their commercial payers, health centers do not have a substantial commercially insured patient base from which to draw. Evidence abounds that the traditional response by physicians and other providers to reduced Medicaid or Medicare payments has been to restrict or reduce the number of publicly-insured patients they serve, often accompanied by a reduction in the amount of indigent care they provide as well.

Because of the shortage of commercial payments, health centers have three options if Medicaid, their largest third party payer, does not cover the cost of providing care to its beneficiaries. They can (1) reduce health care services or reduce the number of health care access points, (2) close their doors entirely—likely resulting in communities having little or no access to primary health care services—or (3) cover Medicaid shortfalls with their PHSA grants intended to defray the cost of caring for the uninsured.

Ensuring the adequacy of payments under Medicaid, regrettably, is not a new issue for health centers. It in fact has been an ongoing concern since the 1990s, during which the relationship between health centers and Medicaid experienced significant challenges as a result of the increased use of Section 1115 waivers in many states. In most cases throughout this period, the ability of health centers to care for Medicaid and uninsured patients was severely damaged when Medicaid payments were cut to only a fraction of the cost of providing care. Moreover, in many of those states, other providers refused to participate or limited their care to only a few Medicaid patients, leaving health centers as one of the few remaining sources of primary and preventive care to this population.

One of the states in which health centers were most impacted during this period was Tennessee. In 1998, the certified public accounting firm of Goldstein, Golub, Kessler and Company (GGK) examined the impact of low-Medicaid payments on health centers in the state under the TennCare program. In GGK's study they found that, while the number of TennCare visits to health centers increased, the gap between revenues and costs per TennCare visit widened, resulting in significant revenue losses for health centers.

By 1996, Tennessee's health centers were losing almost $28 per TennCare patient visit. This created an unfunded gap in reimbursement that forced health centers to cover these losses out of their PHS Act grants. The result was a reduction in the number of uninsured persons receiving care at Tennessee's health centers, and the virtual elimination of all "supplemental" services, including health and nutrition education, parenting classes and community outreach—all of which have been proven highly effective in improving the overall health of patients.

Increasingly, health centers today continue face many of the same challenges with 1115 waivers as they did in the 1990s. Originally created to allow states to try innovative health care approaches, many recently approved waivers have instead been used to limit benefits, increase cost sharing, and reduce enrollment. In some cases, Medicaid provider payments have been cut dramatically, causing other providers to severely limit or end their participation in Medicaid, and leaving health centers—whose mandate is to serve everyone regardless of ability to pay—as one of the few remaining sources of primary and preventive care to this population. If states are permitted to cut Medicaid payments to health centers under these waivers, their ability to care for both Medicaid-covered and uninsured patients would be severely damaged. For these reasons, health centers believe strongly that Medicaid waivers should be approved only if they "promote the objectives of" Medicaid, and do not erode the program's ability to provide comprehensive services to beneficiaries.

As Congress begins to consider reforms to Medicaid, it will be important for lawmakers to appreciate the integral role of health centers and other core safety net providers in Medicaid, and ensure that these providers are adequately paid for the reasonable costs of health care they provide to enrollees. We look forward to continuing to work with Congress in these efforts.

The Importance of Ensuring Future Health Centers Success

Health centers have successfully stood the test of time over the past four decades, not only because they are rooted in the communities they serve, but because of their attention to continuous quality improvement and technical assistance. Since 2002, health centers have expanded to serve an additional 4 million people, adding approximately 3,000 clinicians and several thousand other staffers at centers across the country. With hundreds of new health centers, staff and patients, it is imperative that health centers, whether brand new or established, receive the technical assistance and training required to successfully expand to provide high quality care.

NACHC and State and Regional Primary Care Associations (S/R PCAs) remain fully committed to and engaged in technical assistance activities with health centers. We have long recognized that the success of the program—and current and future expansion initiatives—depends on the ability of health centers to carry out the requirements of the statute and program expectations.

While HRSA has restructured the availability of technical assistance through its project officers, and decreased funding available for on-site assistance for many new centers, HRSA has been able to help health centers plan and implement effective expansion strategies through a cooperative agreement with NACHC and grants to S/R PCAs,. NACHC and the PCAs also conduct trainings for health center staff regarding financial management, clinical practice guidelines, regulatory and legal requirements and consumer board trainings. NACHC also assists communities seeking to apply for new health center funding to meet the federal requirements of the grant.

I am very pleased to report that, over the past few years, NACHC has dramatically increased the frequency and types of education, training and technical assistance it provides. Indeed, since the beginning of the expansion initiative, NACHC has conducted 44 health center grant proposal trainings, some in cooperation with the Bureau of Primary Health Care, PCAs and other organizations, and involving over 3000 individuals interested in starting a health center. In addition to onsite trainings conducted at our two annual conferences, NACHC has also conducted trainings in 12 states. We average 300 technical assistance calls a month. We have also held six onsite orientations for new health centers, and six new start teleconference sessions, providing training for approximately 1100 individuals who are on the staffs and boards of the newly-funded health centers in their communities.

Additionally, NACHC has conducted 35 new health center medical director orientation sessions, providing intensive training to over 1100 medical directors representing 1000 health centers, since 2001. Over this same period of time, our clinical team has also conducted quality management trainings for approximately 720 health centers and their clinicians. NACHC also provides trainings and technical assistance on other key aspects of health center operations, including board governance, financial management, corporate compliance, and strategic business planning. We stand ready to continue our activities in all of these areas to ensure that health centers can build on their record of success over the past 40 years and in this current expansion effort.

Conclusion

Health centers appreciate the unwavering support of Congress for the program over the past four decades. In the past 40 years, health centers have produced a return on the federal investment in the program, by providing access to care and a health care home to millions of patients in medically-underserved communities across the country. Because Congress has continued to reaffirm the core elements of the program; that health centers are open to all, run and controlled by the community, located in high need medically-underserved areas, and provide comprehensive primary and preventive services, the program has successfully faced challenges posed by our ever-changing health care system. On behalf of health centers across the country, their staffs, and the patients they serve, we stand ready to work with you to ensure that health centers continue to provide a health care home for everyone who needs their care. Thank you once again and I would be happy to entertain questions from the committee.

Mr. WHITFIELD. Thank you, Mr. Hawkins.

And Dr. Goetcheus, you are recognized for your opening statement. And be sure and turn your microphone on.

TESTIMONY OF A. JANELLE GOETCHEUS

Ms. GOETCHEUS. Thank you for holding these hearings. Thank you for the opportunity to share today.

I am Janelle Goetcheus. I am the Medical Director of Unity Health Care, which is a federally qualified health center here in Washington. Unity operates a large number of community health centers throughout DC, last year seeing over 55,000 individual patients, representing 240,000 patient visits.

Unity began in 1985 as a health care for the homeless project. And a lot we did here in DC was to place health services directly in the shelters. One of those shelters is just a few blocks away from here at 2nd and D. I think some of the committee members have been there to visit, and we would welcome any others who would want to. A thousand people in one building. We have a health service that runs 6 days a week. It is constantly busy. We have another outreach van with a medical team that goes along Pennsylvania Avenue and some of the parks in the adjacent area looking for homeless folks who need access into health care.

But through the years, we have spread into community health centers throughout the District. And what we have known is it was more than just a doctor's office visit that we needed to provide. We needed to provide a comprehensive set of services, wrap-around services, and so we include mental health and dental and pharmacy. And one of the most important ones is social work. I often say, as a physician, I could never practice without social workers with me. For example, this week, I was with a person who came in who had cancer and was also mentally ill. And I needed to work with a social worker myself to try to get Medicaid for that person in order that I could get chemotherapy for them.

I guess, if anything I would like to share today, and I have heard it here today, is in terms of the quality of the health care that happens in these community health services. I really do think it is equal to any care that you would get in any other place of choice. One of the things that has helped has been these collaboratives, and you have heard some mention of that today.

We participate in a diabetic collaborative. What that means is if a patient comes in to see me who has diabetes, they don't just see me as a primary care provider, they also see the nurse care manager who sits with the patient, teaches them about their illnesses, and helps them set goals for themselves. And we have, and the Bureau of Primary Health Care, has the outcomes related to these initiatives and really can show that we have decreased hospitalizations, decreased emergency room, and decreased all of the complications that diabetes can bring, the early amputations, the early dialysis.

Another great source of help has been the National Health Corps, and I think you would hear this from all of us at the table. We have, for instance, in some of the poorest areas here in DC, we have six health services out there. All of them have National Health Corps physicians. Two of those have been out today making home visits in some of the housing projects, accessing elderly people who otherwise never would have health care.

We also multiply. We take the Federal dollars and we multiply them in various ways. For example, United Health Care this year gave us a $1 million grant, and it will be a multi-year grant to establish improved care at some of our community health centers in these areas. NIH has also been a great partner. They provide care not only on our specialists but also access patients into their own campus. Volunteers also help us. We look forward to hopefully further legislation that would allow the Federal tort to cover volunteer physicians, especially specialists that we often have a great deal of difficulty finding.

We face lots of challenges. You have heard today in terms of the base funding issues, we have benefited by the expanded grants that have come. What we have done from one of our grants is we have gone into the jail, because here in DC, there are over 50 people a day who are coming out of DC jail into the community and another 2,400 that are coming from Federal prisons around the Nation and coming back into the District, and we are trying to connect those folks into ongoing primary health care.

But I think most of all what we do is bring hope to people, not only good primary care, but we bring hope. One of those I think most often of is my friend Robert who I met not very far from here one night, a very cold night, and they were standing around a barrel. And they had built a fire with just some papers to try to keep warm, a group of men. He had a blood pressure of 190 over 135, which is dangerously high, and he is a 54-year-old gentleman. He had worked day labor most of his life and had gotten to that age and couldn't do the heavy lifting anymore, and so he was homeless. But now, instead of around that fire barrel, he was able to move into his own apartment. So I think these community health centers bring good primary care, but they bring hope and they bring hope to many, many Roberts around this Nation.

Thank you.

[The prepared statement of A. Janelle Goetcheus follows:]

PREPARED STATEMENT OF A. JANELLE GOETCHEUS, CHIEF MEDICAL OFFICER UNITY HEALTH CARE, INC.

Good afternoon, my name is Dr. Janelle Goetcheus, Chief Medical Officer of Unity Health Care, Inc. (Unity), Washington, D.C., a Federally Qualified Health Center (FQHC) that operates a large network of health centers which provided health care services to 55,500 patient in 2004, generating over 240,000 patient encounters.

It is a privilege to testify before this Sub-Committee and I thank you Mr. Chairman for the opportunity to do so.

I have over 20 years of experience serving the medically underserved in Washington, D.C., and I wish to speak to you today about the unique value of a community health center in addressing the health care needs of the medically underserved. Let me first tell you about Unity, and the people we serve. Unity began as a private non-profit with funds from the Robert Wood Johnson/Pew Charitable Trust providing health care services to homeless persons. In 1987 we were one of the first federally funded programs under the Stewart B. McKinney Homeless Assistance Act. Over time we expanded our services to include provision of health services in neighborhood/community settings. Today we are the recipient of federal grants under the Community Health Center Consolidated Act, with grants to serve fixed populations in community health centers, homeless persons and we also receive a school based health grant.

Unity provides primary health care services, mental health services, case management, pharmacy, dental, WIC and HIV/Hep-C services throughout the eight (8) wards of the District of Columbia. We do this in fixed sites, homeless shelters, and outreach mobile vans. We have a total of 31 access points throughout our Citywide network.

Of the approximately 55,500 persons served by Unity in 2004 over:

- 75% of them were at 200% or lower of the Federal Poverty Level, most of them were actually 100% or below,
- 74% were uninsured
- 16% were recipients of Medicaid
- 10% Medicare and other
- of our total population served 21% were homeless (on the streets or in shelters)

Of the homeless persons we see approximately:

- 36% are substance abusers
- 19% have mental health issues; much higher percentage for women
- 16% are dually diagnosed
- 20% are veterans, and
- 12% are person living with HIV/Aids.

The ethnic make up of Unity's population is as follows:

- 77% are African American
- 18% are Latino
- 4% other
- 21% are best served by a language other than English.

I share these statistics only to point out that health centers are adept at cultural competence, able to recognize the unique needs of their patients, address them in their own language and culture, and thus remove barriers to care that are often present when serving a mixed racial, ethnic and low income population.

It is important to recognize that health centers provide comprehensive primary health care. This federal requirement to provide comprehensive services enables patients to have the majority of their health care needs addressed in a one stop setting. The comprehensive nature of the care provided goes far beyond a doctors visit. My role as a provider in the health process is important, but I could not practice medicine without the support of a myriad of other providers/services that go into this healing process. Patients we serve have a host of problems, beyond chronic illness. Social workers are an essential part of the provision of health care in a community health center. They assist the provider with arranging for entitlements, and in some cases housing, since over 20% of our patients are homeless, or living in shelters, and many of them suffer from chronic illnesses. As a primary care provider, I often rely on the psychiatrist or mental health worker on staff to link that patient to them so that they can begin to address underlying problems that often go much deeper than the initial presenting symptom. Our patients experience trauma, domestic violence, a family facing eviction, a person with a cocaine addition, a grieving mother; all of these issues can be addressed in a comprehensive manner within a community health center setting.

As the Bureau of Primary Health Care (BPHC) increasingly encourages health center grantees to participate in the Disease Collaboratives, the role of comprehensive health care, and coordinated care management is further emphasized. The Disease Collaboratives are a model of care that places the patient at the center of the care, and he/she is supported in their goal of self-management by a Care Management Team often consisting of a nurse care manager, a social worker, the provider, and other support personnel as needed, such as mental health therapist, pharmacist and speciality providers, i.e. ophthalmologist, podiatrist, in the case of diabetes.

The Chronic Disease Collaboratives nationally have shown that even an indigent and hard to manage population can still generate good health outcomes and improve health status if the care is provided in a coordinated manner. The community health center is the ideal location for the implementation of these Disease Collaboratives because most of the services are on site and the support offered by the overall care team goes far beyond the type of care that an individual physician could provide alone. The clinical data collected through these Disease Collaboratives substantiates the effectiveness of this model of care.

Patients who participate in this model of care have expressed their satisfaction with it, and many for the first time are taking ownership of their health status and realize that their own self involvement, and reliance on support from the care management provided between physician appointments plays a crucial role in their health status.

Unity Has in addition, to the care management structure outlined above, launched its own initiative called "open access" or "same day appointment". This process again calls for a radical re-design of the traditional doctors office visit. A pilot program, with guidance from the Institute for Health Care Improvement (IHI), Unity staff and providers are accommodating patients within 24 hours of their request for care. Traditionally patients requesting care would call up and unless it was an emergency, would be given an appointment on the next available opening which could be weeks or months away. The theory behind "same day access" is to "do today's work today", to address the needs of the patient immediately, and to reduce waste and lost time both for the patient and the staff of the health center. This initiative is now operative in three (3) of Unity's major sites with plans to expand it to the whole network over time.

I point this initiative out as another example of the creativity and adaptability of health centers in addressing the needs of their community, as well as pointing out that health centers are in the forefront of the provision of state of the art health care.

Health Centers are extremely creative in their ability to generate revenues to address the ever increasing number of uninsured and working poor who are coming through their doors. We multiply the Federal dollars made available through the federal grant.

Unity like all other Community Health Centers faces this challenge on a daily basis. We must constantly insure that our ability to survive as a private non-profit is essential, so that we can continue to remain faithful to our mission, a mission "to provide health care to all regardless of ability to pay". Unity currently participates in a District of Columbia sponsored Alliance program, which is essentially a local sponsored uncompensated care pool for uninsured patients under 200% of poverty. We rely on Medicaid, and a vital component of the Medicaid program for us, and for all health centers is the Prospective Payment System (PPS). The PPS system is a method which enables health centers to be compensated for the care they provide to Medicaid patients at a reasonable rate of reimbursement. In a time of budget crunch at the Federal and State levels it is important that the PPS system remains in place for the viability of health centers.

While we are extremely grateful for the President's Five Year Initiative to expand access to care through Community Health Centers it is also important to point out that Unity's base grant has remained stagnant for almost five (5) years. The President's Initiative increases access through "new starts" and "new access points" but does not provide for any base adjustment to existing grantees like Unity, whose numbers of uninsured are rising. Unity like most health centers is creative in building partnerships with other entities, hospitals, health care institutions and corporations to support the strategic interests of their mission. One such partnership of which Unity is extremely proud is our partnership with United Health Care (United), Minnesota. This joint venture results in an annual investment of $1,000,000 over several years by United to one of Unity's health centers to develop a "Center of Excellence" where the model of care management can be implemented in treating several chronic diseases, such as diabetes, cardio-vascular, and asthma, as well as the development of systems to insure improved outcomes in the area of pre-natal care. This "Center of Excellence" drawn from many of the concepts of the Institute for Health Care Improvement (IHI) will serve as a model for further expansion of the concept throughout Unity. Without the financial support of United Health Care, Inc. Unity could not from its existing revenue undertake such a broad based initiative.

For over twenty years it has been my privilege to serve the patients who come to our health centers. I am grateful for how they challenge us, and for the trust they place in us. I have also been privilege to work alongside a committed group of health care professionals, physicians, nurse practitioners, physician assistants, specialists, nurses and social workers. Their commitment to Unity and indeed to the health center movement nationwide is the soul of our success. Many of these professionals come to us through the National Health Service Corps (NHSC) or the Corps Loan Re-Payment Program. This is a vital cog in the machine of recruitment and retention for our health centers. At Unity we witness young African American physicians returning to their neighborhoods giving back to the very people who are their neighbors. Their willingness to come to Unity, often for salaries much less than could get in the commercial market, is another example of the unique role that health centers play in the community, because of their ability to attract such dedicated, committed professionals.

I thank you again for allowing me to testify before you Sub-Committee and I am available to answer any questions.

Mr. WHITFIELD. Thank you, Dr. Goetcheus.

And Mr. Manifold, thank you for joining us. As you can tell, our schedule is so chaotic around here, we do appreciate your coming in. I introduced you earlier, but I am going to call on Dr. Shi to go on and make his statement, and then we will go back to you.

Would you turn your microphone on?

TESTIMONY OF LEIYU SHI

Mr. SHI. Thank you, Mr. Chairman. Thank you, members of the subcommittee for inviting me to testify at your hearing, a review of community health centers: issues and opportunities.

My name is Leiyu Shi. I am a faculty member of the Johns Hopkins Bloomberg School of Public Health. I am also co-director of the Johns Hopkins Primary Care Policy Center for the under-served populations.

For the past 15 years, I have conducted research related to various aspects of community health centers. Today, I would like to share with you some of my and our team's research work related to the role of health centers in improving health care access, quality, and outcome for the Nation's vulnerable populations, particularly the uninsured and racial/ethnic minorities.

Due to time constraints, I will highlight the findings in my presentation and the PowerPoint slides provide the specifics of the findings. Data from which these studies were conducted come from a variety of sources, including that regularly submitted by the federally qualified health centers, regular surveys targeting health centers, new data collection by myself or our research team, and also existing national surveys. The published studies are listed at the end of the handouts and are available upon request.

I would like to start by highlighting the profile of health center patients. Those are in part one of the handouts.

Health center patients are predominantly racial/ethnic minorities. Over 64 percent of those are minorities. Health centers rely heavily on Medicaid funding. Indeed, Medicaid is the single most important funding for health centers for the past 14 years. Health centers are primary care safety net providers for the uninsured, as over 41 percent of health center users are uninsured. They are also primary care safety net providers for the poor, as over 65 percent of health center users are below the Federal poverty line.

Health center patients are sicker than patients seen in any other settings in the country, except emergency rooms. I would like to give some examples of research comparing access to primary health care between health center patients and patients seen in other settings. Those are in part two of the power point handouts.

Among the uninsured patients, those seen by health centers are more likely to have usual source of care than those seen in any other places, 97.5 percent versus 64.9 percent. Health center uninsured patients also have more doctor visits than uninsured patients seen elsewhere, 56 percent versus 33.3 percent with four or more visits per year. Health center patients even outperform nationally privately insured patients on certain access indicators. For example, 97.4 percent health center uninsured and 99.3 percent health center Medicaid patients have usual source of care compared to 91.2 percent nationally privately insured with usual source of care. Over 54 percent of health center uninsured and 65 percent health center Medicaid patients have four or more visits per year compared to 55 percent of nationally privately insured patients with four or more doctor visits per year.

I would like to now provide examples of research comparing access to preventive health care between health center patients and patients seen elsewhere. Those are in part three of the handouts. In terms of cancer screening, pap tests among health center females remain significantly higher than females below 200 percent Federal poverty line in the Nation. Mammography screening among health center females remains significantly higher than the females below 200 percent Federal poverty line in the Nation. Health center diabetic patients use more preventive services, including eye exam, foot exam, flu shot, than diabetic patients nationwide. Health center uninsured and Medicaid adults are more likely to receive health promotion counseling, including smoking, alcohol, exercise, diet, drugs, STDs, than U.S. Medicaid and uninsured patients seen elsewhere.

Let us turn to examples of research comparing quality of health care between health center patients and patients seen elsewhere. Those are in part four of the slides. Health center Medicaid patients are significantly less likely to be hospitalized for potentially avoidable conditions than those obtaining care elsewhere. Health centers patients receive comparable or even better quality primary care services than managed care HMO patients, especially in the comprehensiveness of services provided and the continuity of care.

Finally, I would like to summarize that the above examples of research indicate that health centers provide better access to and quality of care for the Nation's uninsured and low-income minorities than elsewhere for the same vulnerable groups. Their continuous support is critical to the Nation's uninsured and low-income individuals. Providing basic primary health care services to all is a valued national health policy objective.

Thank you very much.

[The prepared statement of Leiyu Shi follows:]

PREPARED STATEMENT OF LEIYU SHI, CO-DIRECTOR, JOHNS HOPKINS PRIMARY CARE POLICY CENTER FOR UNDERSERVED POPULATIONS, JOHNS HOPKINS UNIVERSITY BLOOMBERG SCHOOL OF PUBLIC HEALTH

Distinguished representatives, dear ladies and gentlemen, thank you for inviting me to testify at your hearing titled "a review of community health centers: issues and opportunities."

My name is Leiyu Shi. I am a faculty member from the Johns Hopkins Bloomberg School of Public Health. I am also Co-Director of the Johns Hopkins Primary Care Policy Center for the Underserved Populations. I have a doctorate in public health and masters in public administration and business administration. For the past 15 years, I have conducted research related to various aspects of community health centers. Today I would like to share with you some of my and our team's research work related to the role of health centers in improving access, quality, and outcome for the nation's vulnerable populations particularly the uninsured and racial/ethnic minorities. Due to time constrain, I will highlight the findings in my presentation. The attached power point slides provide the specifics of the findings. Data from which these studies were conducted come from a variety of sources including data regularly submitted by federally qualified health centers (e.g., the Uniform Data System), regular surveys targeting health centers (e.g., Health Center User/Visit Survey), new data collection by myself or our research team (e.g., Sentinel Centers Network Project, numerous surveys of health centers), and existing national surveys (e.g., National Health Interview Survey). The published studies are listed at the end of the slides and are available upon request. Further questions, comments, or discussions can be directly to me through e-mail at lshi@jhsph.edu.

I'd like to start by highlighting the profile of health center patients (see Part I of the power point slides). Health center patients are predominantly racial/ethnic minorities (64%). Health centers rely heavily on Medicaid funding (33%). Health centers are primary care safety-net providers for the uninsured (41%) and the poor (65% below FPL). Health center patients are sicker than patients seen in other settings.

I'd like to give some examples of research comparing access to primary health care between health center patients and patients seen in other settings (see Part II of the power point slides). Among the uninsured patients, those seen by health centers are more likely to have usual source of care than those seen elsewhere (97.5% vs. 64.9%). Health center uninsured patients also have more doctor visits than uninsured patients seen elsewhere (56% vs. 33.3% with 4 or more visits per year). Health center patients even outperform nationally privately insured patients on certain access indicators. For example, 97.4% health center uninsured and 99.3% health center Medicaid patients have usual source of care compared to 91.2% nationally privately insured with usual source of care. Over 54% of health center uninsured and 64.6% of health center Medicaid patients have 4 or more doctor visits per year, compared to 54.9% of nationally privately insured patients with 4 or more doctor visits per year.

I'd like to provide examples of research comparing access to preventive health care between health center patients and patients seen elsewhere (see Part III of the power point slides). In terms of cancer screening, pap tests among health center females remain significantly higher than females below 200% FPL in the nation. Mammography screenings among health center females remain significantly higher than the females below 200% FPL in the nation. Health Center diabetic patients use more preventive services (including eye exam, foot exam, flu shot, pneumovax) than diabetic patients nationwide. Health center uninsured and Medicaid adults are more likely to receive health promotion counseling (including smoking, alcohol, exercise, diet, drugs, STDs) than U.S. Medicaid and uninsured patients).

Let's turn to examples of research comparing quality of health care between health center patients and patients seen elsewhere (see Part IV of the power point slides). Health center Medicaid patients are significantly less likely to be hospitalized for potentially avoidable conditions than those obtaining care elsewhere. Health centers patients receive comparable or even better quality primary care services than managed care (HMO) patients especially in the comprehensiveness of services provided and the continuity of care.

Finally, I'd like to share examples of research comparing outcomes of care between health center patients and patients seen elsewhere (see Part V of the power point slides). Babies born to health center mothers enjoy lower rates of low birth weight than those born elsewhere. There is significantly less racial disparity in low birth weight rate within health centers than within the nation as a whole (3.25 times vs. 5.6 times). Had the health center program become available to all the low-income blacks in this country, 17,107 fewer low birth weight incidences would result annually.

In conclusion, I would like to emphasize that the above examples of research indicate that health centers provide better access to and quality of care for the nation's uninsured and low-income minorities than elsewhere for the same vulnerable groups. Their continual support is critical to the nation's uninsured and low-income individuals if providing basic primary health care services to all is a valued national health policy objective.

Mr. WHITFIELD. Thank you, Dr. Shi.

And at this time, Mr. Manifold, as you are aware, this is an investigative hearing, and I would like to swear you in for your testimony.

[Witness sworn.]

Mr. WHITFIELD. Thank you very much, and you may proceed with your opening statement.

TESTIMONY OF RODERICK V. MANIFOLD

Mr. MANIFOLD. Thank you for your indulgence, Mr. Chairman, members of the committee.

Thank you for inviting me to testify before you today about Central Virginia Health Services, our community health center in central Virginia. I am Rod Manifold, and I am the CEO of CVHS. Our health center really got started back in 1968 when a lady named Buelah Wiley slumped down in a chair at the local Community Action Program offices and said, "We should not have to drive an hour and a half one way to take a child to see the doctor." From that moment, community activities began that culminated in the establishment in 1970 of Central Virginia Community Health Center, now called Central Virginia Health Services.

Today, our health center is a 10-site family of health centers serving 18 counties and cities that are located from the northern neck of Virginia to the city of Petersburg, south to the North Carolina State line and west as far as Albemarle County and Charlottesville. Central Virginia Health Services is the oldest community health center organization in Virginia and is celebrating its 35th year of operation in 2005. Last year, Central Virginia served over 34,000 people, and it is still operated as it was in 1970 by a board of directors made up of community members that are committed to its mission. In fact, 63 percent of our board members are users of our services. This community representation tempered with the responsibility for the mission of the entire health center is one of the hallmarks of the health center movement.

As in the 1970's, poverty and lack of access to care are still primary reasons for the existence of Central Virginia and the many other health centers around Virginia and around the country. Lack of income, racial disparities, and lack of access are all reasons why health centers are needed in central Virginia. In the Central Virginia Health Services sites in 2004, more than half of our patients were minorities, 30 percent were below the Federal poverty guideline, and 31 percent were completely uninsured.

As you may know, community health centers do charge fees to all of these patients. These are not free clinics, because Congress in its wisdom set them up to collect fees on a sliding scale basis from each and every one of our patients. All consumers of our services participate in funding their community health center based upon their ability to pay. It gives them a kind of ownership of the health center in their community, and it clearly states to them that these services have a value.

In recent years, under the President's initiative to expand health centers, Central Virginia, like many other health centers around the country, has been able to expand services and add additional access points for care in many communities. We competed for and received a grant for a new access point in Charles City County that has helped create a totally new health center with medical, dental, and behavioral health services in a county that previously had one part-time doctor serving the community only three half-days per week and no dentist or psychologist. Additionally, we receive grants to expand medical capacity in two existing health centers, and we also received a grant to add dental services in a health center that was previously providing only medical services. All of these additional services and sites would not have been possible without the HRSA grants awarded under the President's initiative.

In addition to thanking this subcommittee for its support of the expansion of the program, I would be remiss if I didn't also discuss the critical importance of the Medicaid program to our health center. We respect that your committee has a very difficult challenge in looking at reductions in the Medicaid program. That being said, we do want to make one thing very clear. The prospective payment system that Congress has given to health centers because of our unique place in the safety net is very important to health centers. We know that our patients in that safety net will be our patients regardless of what sort of payment methodology is created here. Obviously, if the PPS was tinkered with, health centers could suffer greatly. In addition, if Medicaid primary care benefits are reduced, our patients will still need those services. We will just have to use the Federal grant, which is designed to serve the many uninsured patients in our centers, to subsidize the Medicaid program and its patients.

In conclusion, Mr. Chairman and members of the subcommittee, I appreciate the opportunity to discuss our work at Central Virginia Health Services, and we appreciate the recent expansion opportunities provided to all health centers. We also stand ready to work with you as you debate changes in the Medicaid program that may have a significant impact on our operations and the patients we serve.

Thank you for your time, and I am happy to answer any questions you may have.

[The prepared statement of Roderick V. Manifold follows:]

PREPARED STATEMENT OF RODERICK V. MANIFOLD, EXECUTIVE DIRECTOR, CENTRAL VIRGINIA HEALTH SERVICES, INC.

In 1968 a staff member named Beulah Wiley of the Community Action Program in Cumberland County, Virginia returned from taking a child to the doctor at the University of Virginia Medical Center. She reportedly slumped down in a chair at the CAP offices and said, "We should not have to drive an hour and a half, one way, to take a child to see the doctor." From that moment community activities (and I emphasize that word community) began that culminated in the establishment in 1970 of Central Virginia Community Health Center, located in Buckingham County and serving three counties.

Today that health center has grown to a ten-site family of health centers serving 18 counties and cities that are located from the Northern Neck of Virginia to the city of Petersburg, south to the North Carolina state line and west as far as Albemarle County and Charlottesville. Central Virginia Health Services, as it is called today, is the oldest community health center organization in Virginia and is celebrating its 35th year of operation in 2005. Last year Central Virginia served a diverse population of over 34,000 people in rural and urban sites across its many community service areas. It is still operated, as it was in 1970, by a board of directors made up of community members that are committed to its mission. In fact, as many of you may know, at least 51% of the board members of a community health center must be consumers of the health center's services. Last year, 63% of our board members were users of our services. This community representation tempered with responsibility for the mission of the entire health center is one of the hallmarks of the health center movement. Being patients as well as leaders of the policy-setting board makes our members the best possible representatives of their communities and of the thousands of patients we serve.

As in the 1970's, poverty and lack of access to care are still primary reasons for the existence of Central Virginia and the many other health centers around Virginia and around the country. The high poverty rate, severe health care disparities, and the lack of access to the health care system are all reasons why health centers are needed in central Virginia. In the Central Virginia Health Services sites in 2004, for example, more than half (51%) of our patients were minorities, 30% were below the federal poverty guideline, and 31% were completely uninsured. These numbers of high need are not unusual for a community health center. In fact, in one of our urban centers, over 50% of our patients are uninsured and fully 70% are below the federal poverty guideline.

As you may know, community health centers do charge fees to all of these patients. These are not free clinics, because Congress in its wisdom set them up to collect fees on a sliding scale basis from each and every one of our patients. All consumers of our services participate in funding their community health center based upon their ability to pay. It gives them a kind of "ownership" of the health center in their community, and it clearly states to them that these services have a value. Last year Central Virginia Health Services collected from our various payer sources (not including the federal grant we receive to assist the uninsured patients), 24% of our patient income from private insurance companies, 30% from Medicaid, 20% from Medicare, and 26% directly from patients' payments. As an example of those patient payments, we have a collection rate of over 95% from our Medicare patients for the services they receive from our providers. While these numbers are not the same in every health center, virtually all health centers work to develop a broad spectrum of payer sources, in addition to the HRSA grant.

In recent years, under the President's initiative to expand health centers, Central Virginia, has been able to expand services and add additional access points for care in many communities. We competed for and received a grant for a new access point in Charles City County, a jurisdiction with a minority population of over 75%. This grant helped to create a totally new health center with medical, dental and behavioral health services in a county that previously had one part-time private doctor serving the community only three half days per week and no dentists or psychologists. Additionally we received grants to expand medical capacity in two existing health centers, and we also received a grant to add dental services in a health center that was previously providing only medical services. All of these additional services and sites would not have been possible without the HRSA grants awarded under the President's Initiative and funded by Congress. And these grants have stimulated private foundations to provide funding for additional services to be provided in several of our existing health centers.

Of perhaps even more compelling interest to this subcommittee and your full committee, are some issues related to Medicaid and Medicare. Frankly, as a community health center director, I worry about these two major payer sources for our patients. Remember that we health centers are the true safety net providers of primary care for many of our nation's most vulnerable citizens. And I mean, we really are working in the frayed bottom of that safety net. We live day to day, and we get very concerned when Congress begins to discuss cuts to the Medicaid program. We respect that your committee and the Medicaid Commission have a very difficult challenge in looking at reductions in the Medicaid program. That being said, we do want to make one thing very clear: the prospective payment system (PPS) that Congress has given to health centers because of our unique place in the safety net is very, very important to health centers. We know that our patients in that safety net will be our patients regardless of what sort of payment methodology is created here. Obviously, if the PPS was tinkered with, health centers could suffer greatly. In addition, if Medicaid primary care benefits are reduced, our patients will still need those services. We will just have to use the federal grant, which is designed to serve the many uninsured patients in our centers, to "subsidize" the Medicaid program and its patients. Furthermore, if Medicaid eligibility limits are lowered, and more patients are moved off the Medicaid rolls, we in health centers will still serve those patients, only they will then join the ranks of the uninsured. Reductions in benefits and/or eligibility levels for Medicaid will be a real double whammy to health centers and their patients, and could well bring about drastic reductions in programs and services—exactly the opposite of the goal for the President's Initiative. At Central Virginia, our providers and staff know these patients very well, and we know that they will look to us for their care, regardless of whether they have Medicaid or not.

Also of interest to this subcommittee, of course, is the Medicare Part D program. The provision of pharmaceuticals to Medicare patients will be the largest contributor to better health outcomes for our health center Medicare patients since the inception of the Medicare program itself. We look forward to 2006 and we hope that the development of training and orientation programs and materials for seniors and for us caregivers of seniors will come in time for every Medicare recipient to benefit fully from this new service. We know that CMS and other agencies are working to meet the deadline set by Congress for the initiation of this program. Please know that we in community health centers will do everything possible to assist in this monumental effort, because we truly know how important it is to the health of our individual patients.

I would like to tell you about another part of the community health center story in one of our communities: Farmville and Prince Edward County, Virginia. In the mid-1980's the Piedmont Health District serving these two localities and the surrounding counties had one of the highest infant mortality rates in the Commonwealth of Virginia. In 1985 Central Virginia Health Services, the Virginia Department of Health, and the federal government collaborated to open the Women's Health Center in Farmville. This OB-Gyn practice started small with one physician and a tiny group of support staff. The Health Center for Women and Families, as it is called today, now provides the only obstetric services in this rural community. Our center there has two full time OB-Gyn physicians, one full time family practice physician, and one part time nurse midwife doing deliveries in the local hospital and, along with a full time nurse practitioner, they also provide virtually all of the prenatal care for the community. This is a real success story for Farmville and the surrounding area. While several community hospitals in Virginia have recently closed down their labor and delivery service due to skyrocketing malpractice insurance and other factors, Southside Community Hospital, with our assistance, has been able to not only keep its community obstetric program, but to make it grow and thrive. By the way, the infant mortality rate has gone down over the past twenty years and the community and its families are all the better for that positive outcome.

I would like to close with a story about the first community health center patient in Virginia. Dr. Mike Shepherd, a University of Virginia physician and the first physician of Central Virginia Community Health Center, recounts this story of opening day on the Friday after Thanksgiving in 1970. I have told it many times because I believe it illustrates why health centers are an absolute necessity in many communities around our country. A woman in her eighties was brought to the center by her family on that first day. She was being interviewed by the nurse taking her health history. The nurse asked the woman when was the last time she was seen by a doctor. The woman thought for a few moments and finally said, "Nineteen and twenty-three." And that is why health centers are needed. Here was woman who was not seen by a doctor for nearly 50 years. And, while we don't find many patients these days with such a long time between visits, we do know that we serve people who need us and who would not be seen if it were not for the health center in their communities.

Mr. WHITFIELD. Thank you, Mr. Manifold.

And I would ask all of you, are any of you familiar with some community health centers over the last couple of years that have gone into bankruptcy or have gone out of operation? Are any of you aware of any that have gone out of business?

Mr. HAWKINS. On a national level, Mr. Chairman, what I can tell you is I have not seen data for the last couple of years, but I have no reason to suspect it is different from the data I have seen for the previous 10 years. In any given year, three to five health centers will have their grant pulled. They will be defunded. They will be folded into another center. An effort is always made by, I am going to call them the feds, HRSA to keep the services going when an existing health center runs into trouble. But that is three to five out of 1,000. So that is a failure rate of less than 1 percent. I have never seen it exceed 1 percent.

Mr. WHITFIELD. And they are basically folded in with another when that occurs?

Mr. HAWKINS. Most often. I think it is quite rare when HRSA has pulled the resources completely out of the community, but they do insist that centers be well managed.

Mr. WHITFIELD. Right. Now patients pay on a sliding scale. Some do not have to pay anything, and others pay full price. Those of you who operate a center, could you tell me the range of prices that are paid per visit by a patient? From zero to what?

Mr. MANIFOLD. Well, we established these sets of charges based on the statute that basically sets it at the cost of doing business the usual and customary in the community. So you could be, in some communities, as much as $50 or $60 or $70 a visit for someone who is able to pay the full charge.

Mr. WHITFIELD. So if I come in and I am over the poverty level, and say I am at 200 percent of the poverty level, and I come in Petersburg, Virginia to the clinic, what would I be expected to pay per visit?

Mr. MANIFOLD. If you are over 200 percent of the poverty level?

Mr. WHITFIELD. Yes.

Mr. MANIFOLD. You would pay the full charge, whatever it is in that particular community.

Mr. WHITFIELD. So it would be, maybe, $50 or $60?

Mr. MANIFOLD. It could be, yes. I can't tell you right off the top of my head what it is. Part of it depends on your health and what sort of services you receive at that time.

Mr. WHITFIELD. Okay. So it does depend on the service? It is not just the one fee.

Mr. MANIFOLD. Just like any other health care institution, yes.

Mr. WHITFIELD. Okay. Now I have heard some discussion about the President's budget and even though he is requesting more money for the centers, people are concerned that because each center receives a grant each year, that even though more money being available and wanting to create more new centers that the existing centers are a little bit concerned about whether or not they are going to continue to receive their grant each year. Is that a concern or is that not a concern?

Mr. HAWKINS. Nationally, I think, Mr. Chairman, every health center must go through a competing grant renewal process every, what is it, Rod, 3 years or 5?

Mr. MANIFOLD. Yes, three to five.

Mr. HAWKINS. Three to 5 years depending on how good their record is and how well they are operated. The best operated ones perhaps every 5 years. They do have to submit documentation and annual audits, et cetera, every year. I will let the actual health center folks answer, but I will tell you what we have heard from health centers is not so much that they are concerned about losing their current grant, it is that the grant doesn't keep pace with the increased costs.

Mr. WHITFIELD. Okay.

Mr. HAWKINS. Health center cost increases on a per-patient basis are among the lowest in the health care system, usually about 4 percent a year, and that is over the last 8 years.

Mr. WHITFIELD. And what is the maximum grant that one can receive?

Mr. HAWKINS. There is no ceiling on that. Although not on a formula basis, it is done often related to per-patient cost or per-uninsured patient——

Mr. WHITFIELD. Well, what grants do you all receive? The ones here.

Mr. MANIFOLD. Well, at Central Virginia, we have added various sites over the years from that original site in 1970.

Mr. WHITFIELD. Right.

Mr. MANIFOLD. And so each time that we have been able to add a site, we have been able to get additional funding for that site, which then stays with it?

Mr. WHITFIELD. How much?

Mr. MANIFOLD. Well, I can tell you that in 1995, we were getting $250,000 per year to start a new health center site. Now you must provide more services. You must provide dental, behavioral health——

Mr. WHITFIELD. But do you have an overall figure of what your center receives?

Mr. MANIFOLD. What Central Virginia receives?

Mr. WHITFIELD. Yes.

Mr. MANIFOLD. We receive $5.2 million in Central Virginia.

Mr. WHITFIELD. Okay. Okay.

Mr. MANIFOLD. It is about 34 percent of our operation——

Mr. WHITFIELD. Okay. What about you, Ms. Sibilsky, in Michigan?

Ms. SIBILSKY. I am a primary care association.

Mr. WHITFIELD. Right.

Ms. SIBILSKY. We are not a health center, specifically.

Mr. WHITFIELD. Oh, you are not?

Ms. SIBILSKY. No.

Mr. WHITFIELD. So——

Ms. SIBILSKY. We are a Statewide association that works with health centers.

Mr. WHITFIELD. So you don't receive any grants?

Ms. SIBILSKY. We do receive a grant to do technical assistance and support to health centers as well as going to communities to help them get ready to be able to provide that primary care.

Mr. WHITFIELD. How much is your grant that you receive?

Ms. SIBILSKY. We receive about $625,000 for the technical assistance component.

Mr. WHITFIELD. Okay. Okay. And what about you, Dr. Goetcheus?

Ms. GOETCHEUS. I was just getting the answer to that, $6.4 million is what we——

Mr. WHITFIELD. $6.4 million.

Ms. GOETCHEUS. [continuing] receive.

Mr. WHITFIELD. Okay.

Ms. GOETCHEUS. Just in regard to what was asked as far as the base funding, we do get concerned. The health care costs for insurance for our folks go up——

Mr. WHITFIELD. Right.

Ms. GOETCHEUS. [continuing] as well as just basic expenses, so we do get very concerned about base funding.

Mr. WHITFIELD. Now I have heard different answers on this question. Can you or can you not spend money on capital projects from the grant money?

Mr. HAWKINS. On acquisition and lease, yes; on construction, modernization, renovation, no.

Mr. WHITFIELD. But on acquisition and lease, yes.

Mr. HAWKINS. Yes.

Mr. WHITFIELD. But for renovation and modernization, no.

Mr. HAWKINS. Any bricks and mortar. If you need to put in an elevator to make the facility ADA compliant, no go.

Mr. WHITFIELD. Okay.

Mr. HAWKINS. If you need to wire the facility for electronic health records, no.

Mr. WHITFIELD. Right.

Mr. HAWKINS. If you need to paint the interior of the facility, you may not use the grant dollars for that purpose. It is prohibited.

Mr. WHITFIELD. Okay.

Mr. HAWKINS. That was stripped from the statute 10 years ago.

Mr. WHITFIELD. Okay. Okay. Now someone made the comment that community health centers provide care for 10 percent of the Medicaid population at a cost of only 1 percent of the total Medicaid dollars. Is that correct?

Mr. HAWKINS. That is correct, Mr. Chairman. Six million people, it is less than $3 billion. The last number I have is $2.5 billion in total Medicaid payments to health centers for approximately 6 million Medicaid recipients. That is under $500 per patient per year for the four visits that Dr. Shi mentioned.

Mr. WHITFIELD. And some of you may have heard in my opening statement I made the comment we have people on Medicare, we have people on Medicaid, and then we have a lot of uninsured who are working who have jobs, but their employer does not provide their health insurance. They are paying taxes for Medicare and taxes for Medicaid, but they can not afford to buy their own health insurance and they maybe do not have a community health center area to visit. So I would ask the question, do you believe that community health centers have the capacity with the right resources available to be the primary health and preventive care providers for the country for the uninsured, let us say? Or is that capability not——

Ms. SIBILSKY. It would be a wonderful model with limitless resources to be able to provide. I believe in the model I worked with modeled for 26 years, comprehensive, primary care, prevention, and community based. It is also a wonderful part of a whole system of care, and that is the way I think we have to look at it, because there are not limitless resources. It is a tremendous model, especially in under-served communities.

Mr. HAWKINS. It is a model for primary care, Mr. Chairman. I have been in it for 35 years, and I don't know that even I, in my ideal world vision, would see health centers even as the primary care provider for all Americans, although there are those who would say that they would only wish that they could get primary care for their family like they have seen delivered at a health center. But for uninsured, for low-income, both publicly insured and uninsured, for isolated rural, for inner city communities, for those working people that you talk about, with or without insurance coverage, every American needs, and Dr. Shi can speak to this, two things for good health, and plus their own thing, and that is insurance coverage to make the care affordable and a health care home, a family doctor who is the organizer of their care. I don't see health centers doing specialty care, doing inpatient hospital, or long-term care, but primary care and being the care manager for each individual, organizing referrals, et cetera, down the road.

Mr. SHI. I just want to add that I do believe that the community health centers are a very well suited model for community-based primary care for all Americans. And many physicians' offices are not equipped to provide enabling services and culturally sensitive care that community health centers are able to provide.

Mr. WHITFIELD. Right. Okay. And you studied them quite a bit. So thank you.

Mr. SHI. Yes.

Mr. WHITFIELD. My time is expired, so I recognize Mr. Stupak.

Mr. STUPAK. Thank you, Mr. Chairman, and thank you all for being here and doing what you do. I have quite a few health centers in my District, and I am always amazed at the work they do on a very, very thin dime.

Why was the brick and mortar stripped out 10 years ago? You said that. Was it alleged abuse within the program or what happened? Because I mean, it seems to be a big issue with health care centers.

Mr. HAWKINS. It is a cautionary tale, and what can happen some time when something is inadvertent and unintentional. In the process of stripping out language that related to the Davis Bacon wage and hour law, which had been in the statute since 1978, the Congress inadvertently, we believe, and certainly even those who were involved in it told us they never intended to strip out the authority for construction, only the language that related to the Davis Bacon law. Unfortunately, what was stripped was all of the construction modernization and expansion language. And attempts to restore that since that time have not been successful.

Mr. STUPAK. Is there opposition from others for——

Mr. HAWKINS. No one opposes restoring the construction authority. The authority for health centers to use even a small portion, no one believes that a big part of the health center funding should go for bricks and mortar. It is patient care dollars. But no one opposes restoring the authority for some portion of that to be used for bricks and mortar. The divide, Mr. Stupak, is literally over whether to restore it without Davis Bacon or with Davis Bacon, and there, unfortunately, quite frankly, I don't think it is a divide up here. It is a divide out there.

Mr. STUPAK. Well, let me ask this question. There are a number of health care centers that have increased significantly in the last few years, and there is an increased likelihood that centers will be located in areas where they are in competition with other health centers and private practitioners. With resources being stretched, what safeguards are used, if you know, in the grant review process, this is really a question I had for HRSA, but I never got to it, to ensure that placement of health centers are in the proper location so that agency gets the best bang for its buck, its Federal dollars? How do you do that? I mean, actually some folks have said we don't want health centers where we have other private practitioners. And is that part of the problem here?

Mr. HAWKINS. It may be in some communities. I remember in south Texas 35 years ago a grave concern among the local private practice physicians at the startup of our health center, they all understood that there was a population that they didn't have the resources to care for. And they were happy to have the health center care for that population. They were deeply concerned about that center then being a place that might encourage people with private insurance to go.

Mr. STUPAK. I see.

Mr. HAWKINS. As time went on, I think all of the private practitioners, in fact, they all donated their time to the facility, they came to see, and I will defer to my colleagues who are out there today.

Mr. STUPAK. Sure, I would be interested to what Dr. Goetcheus thought on that one.

Mr. HAWKINS. They came to see it much more as a benefit than not.

Ms. GOETCHEUS. In terms of DC, the need is so great that two of the new starts that have just come are within a few blocks of one of our health services. The need is so great; we are all very busy. I think——

Mr. STUPAK. Do specialists, though, not want you in the area because you may detract from their patients? Specialists?

Ms. GOETCHEUS. Specialists are hard to obtain, and they are very hard to obtain in terms of accepting Medicaid or here in the District, trying to find those specialists who will accept that kind of insurance. That is why we have brought specialists to our sites. One of the limiting factors has been in terms of the Federal tort for them. For example, we have so many HIV patients, so we have hired two infectious disease physicians to be a part of our staff, because trying to find access otherwise for them with Medicaid or no insurance is very hard.

Mr. STUPAK. It is very difficult. Sure.

Mr. Chairman, if I may, with your permission, the reinstatement of oral health benefits for Medicaid adults, I think every one of our witnesses here this afternoon mentioned adult oral health care and the benefits thereof, and this actually happens to be from Ms. Sibilsky's group. It is a three-page document, and if you don't mind, I would like to place it into the record and—well, it is already in the record. Okay. Great.

But Kim, could you just mention some of the highlights you found? I found this really fascinating. Michigan did it for the first time, and then unfortunately we have to cut it out after being so successful because there is no money there. But you have all mentioned it, and I just want to——

Ms. SIBILSKY. Yes. For a $9.2 million savings in general fund for the State budget, we have done an assessment of inappropriate care in the emergency room, which begins to approach that $9.2 million. When you then look at the Medicaid managed care billings that are addressing the issues that would appropriately be handled within the health centers in their dental component, you get very, very close to the $9.2 million savings. And that doesn't even address how ill people get when they have that primary infection in their mouth: heart disease, diabetes, perinatal health is just directly impacted. I think that it is a service that has been seen to be not a primary care service, but is now being looked at and sadly being looked at so closely because we are in such big trouble with it. I would hope that some day it is seen to be a mandatory service under Medicaid and not an optional service, because it is such a critical need.

Mr. STUPAK. And then I am a little confused, and maybe you can help me on this. From what I have read, the Surgeon General of the United States keeps saying that we don't need this service, the oral health care for folks, or do I have that right? He encourages or discourages it?

Ms. SIBILSKY. I can't speak to that, Mr. Stupak. I am sorry.

Mr. STUPAK. Okay. So in Michigan now, are they getting dental care, the patients?

Ms. SIBILSKY. At this point, under the Medicaid program, only emergency care is being delivered and paid for. For any dental services beyond that to adults that are being delivered in the health centers is being subsidized by the Federal grant as uninsured. So you have Medicaid-covered adults categorized as uninsured for dental services. So the grant is subsidizing Medicaid on those services.

Mr. STUPAK. Okay. I talked about, earlier, rural programs, and I didn't get to ask all of my questions, because I was concerned about the nursing act. I was concerned about the huge cut that we saw in the funds to try to lure specialists to our rural areas or under-served areas. And in those two programs, I think one was cut like $100 million this year and then next year it is going to be $11 million and then that just about wipes about that program. That is the program to attract specialists to our areas. And if we don't fund these programs, what is going to happen to bring your specialists in? You all talk about collaborative efforts you have with other people. Are these specialists volunteering their time, or do they expect some kind of reimbursement, because I just don't see how we are going to continue to do what you are doing as we are expanding the number of health care centers when the programs we have to provide rural health and to recruit physicians and everything else is being severely cut? I mean, Dr. Burgess talked about we need, for doctors, higher reimbursement, but you have got to have doctors there first before you have to worry about reimbursements, and we are not getting the doctors. Am I wrong?

Ms. SIBILSKY. I would like to cite the large amount of volunteerism that is actually happening within the State of Michigan right now. Physicians went into health service for altruistic reasons, and when they feel the intensity of the problem the way that they are feeling it today, they do volunteer. And that is why the Federal torts claims act coverage for free clinics has been very helpful and why extending that into health centers is going to be even more important. The training programs are under siege with the State budgets. For them to be under siege with the Federal budget puts us, once again, right in the middle of the fire. This is not a simple Medicaid issue that we are dealing with. We are under duress on every side. And so the programs you asked about, for example, the rural health outreach program that has helped communities innovate in order to attempt to invent themselves out of these problems through collaborative efforts and outreach efforts. To have those zeroed out is also a very big problem for rural communities.

Mr. STUPAK. Yes, it is about a 70 percent cut.

Mr. Manifold, how about the rural flexibility grant programs? Have you used that? Has that helped? Michigan, right now we have got some high unemployment. We are having some tough times in Michigan, but Virginia seems to be doing a little bit better from what I read in the local papers.

Mr. MANIFOLD. We do not use that program in Virginia, that I know of, not in the health center arena, so I can't speak to that issue.

Mr. STUPAK. That is interesting.

Mr. MANIFOLD. Unless I am not understanding the terminology.

Mr. STUPAK. Well, the rural flexibility grant program actually helps our hospitals in northern Michigan go into the critical access hospitals, which are the smaller hospitals that provide critical access in really remote rural areas, and they get a pretty good reimbursement. And that program actually is one of those that has really been a great help to us, and we see it zeroed out in the budget, so I thought you just might have the same thing.

Mr. MANIFOLD. Yes. Because the critical access hospitals in Virginia are few and far between, many in southwest Virginia, I can't say that our particular arena of health centers in Central Virginia has any connection directly with any critical access hospitals in Virginia.

Mr. HAWKINS. Mr. Stupak, if I could add, though.

Mr. STUPAK. Sure.

Mr. HAWKINS. Across the country, we have heard from health centers who have worked very closely with critical access hospitals in their communities. Health centers help those hospitals keep their doors open. They staff them, especially in the taking evenings and weekends, et cetera, and they have reported. I mean, the affiliation is in partnerships that have developed across the country between health centers and hospitals and especially in rural communities where they are so crucial to one another. They are interdependent. It is heartening to see, because each is helping to keep the other in business for the benefit of the community.

Mr. STUPAK. Sure. One more, if I may.

Dr. Shi, you mentioned in your oral testimony that health center patients receive "comparable or even better quality primary care services than managed care HMO patients, especially in the comprehensiveness of service provided and the continuity of care." When I was asking Mr. Smith the questions there, and even Dr. Duke, they kept talking about other sources of funding. The only other sources of funding I have really seen being pushed is probably managed care or, as you all do, private fundraising to keep you guys open. If we continue to move toward HMOs or managed care, do you feel there will be a decline in the quality of service provided to our patients?

Mr. SHI. Compared to community health centers, I agree. Yes, it is on my page 36 of the handouts. I have the details of that study.

Mr. STUPAK. Okay.

Mr. SHI. It compares HMO with health center patients in terms of the primary care they received from the doctors. And we look at various domains of primary care using our primary care assessment tool. We find that——

Mr. STUPAK. There it is.

Mr. SHI. Yes. If you look at comprehensiveness of services, health centers are rated much higher than HMOs, and the continuity of care, they are also rated higher than HMOs. On the other indicators of primary care quality, they are comparable. And the overall primary care score is also higher among health center patients than among HMOs.

Mr. STUPAK. Thank you. Thank you for the time.

Mr. WHITFIELD. There are a number of areas I want to get into in just a minute here.

On the managed care issue, I know there was some testimony that because managed care pays so little on reimbursement, that the State, I believe, has to make up that difference in the reimbursement to the community health center in most States or all States, is that correct?

Mr. HAWKINS. All States.

Mr. WHITFIELD. Okay. Okay. And so Dr. Shi is making the argument that the managed care, we are underpaying but they are not providing the quality of health care. But on Michigan just a minute, the dental program in Michigan was dropped. That was a decision that the State of Michigan made, and it sounds like it was a short-sighted decision, because they are saving $9.2 million by dropping it, but maybe infection rates have gone up and health care has gone up and so overall Medicaid costs have probably escalated. Is that right?

Ms. SIBILSKY. We are seeing symptoms of that.

Mr. WHITFIELD. Okay. Now I know that there are some loan guarantee programs out there for the community health centers. And maybe you, Ms. Sibilsky, have even made the argument during the 1980's that some changes were made to the community health center program that gave you the flexibility of running it more as a business than as a government entity and that sort of freedom provided you with some innovative opportunities. Would you expand on that a little bit for us?

Ms. SIBILSKY. I believe that much of the value of health centers has been displayed in its ability to be a business and be viable and be managed accordingly. It has spurred innovation to keep us viable. It has also helped us, I believe, to become a bipartisanly supported program.

Mr. WHITFIELD. Right.

Ms. SIBILSKY. Communities, as Mr. Manifold says, and I will yield to him, want to participate in something that they can pay for and receive value.

Mr. WHITFIELD. Right.

Ms. SIBILSKY. And I believe very strongly in those precepts in our program.

Mr. WHITFIELD. Well, you know, one of the frustrating things for me, having been elected to Congress in 1994, we have been talking about trying to address the uninsured program, and I know people go in and out of uninsured status, but we have some areas of the country that have wonderful community health centers, like your area, Mr. Manifold, where more and more people are going to those centers. And then we have other centers that the taxpayers don't have anything. And so we have some people paying taxes, and they have a tremendous program, and others are paying taxes that have nothing. And that is why I was asking this question about using this as a model to be the primary care for the Nation. And I think the consensus was, among this group at least, that you would probably agree with that.

Now let me ask this question. Would you agree if State Medicaid programs individually could use their Medicaid dollars to expand community health centers? I mean, they are already paying a lot of health care providers. Maybe they could get a group together and say won't you provide this service under the community health center umbrella. Would you support that kind of a concept?

Mr. HAWKINS. Mr. Chairman, if it were an allowable use of Medicaid dollars. Although, I suppose, under administrative cost expenses, and I assume what you are talking about is the startup costs for establishing and getting a health center going.

Mr. WHITFIELD. Right. Right.

Mr. HAWKINS. The one big question, then, that would come up is the Federal grants that Mr. Manifold receives, that Dr. Goetcheus' center receives really, if you look at how a health center budget breaks out, and then the patient population by payer source, the Federal grants really truly go to cover care for the uninsured. So I guess the only question left would be, then, would Medicaid be paying for the uninsured? They don't at health centers today.

Mr. WHITFIELD. Right.

Mr. HAWKINS. And there is always a concern. We have heard that from Medicare and Medicaid. We are happy to pay for care for our beneficiaries, but we don't want to be paying for others.

Mr. WHITFIELD. Right. Well, just kind of discussing things here, I read an article not too long ago that General Motors is now paying more for its health care costs than it is for its material for the car or the vehicles that they produce. What would you think about if General Motors could put money into establishing a community health center under all of the Federal guidelines with all of the drug discounts, the tort claim liability protection and whatever, but they had to put the money into it to expand it to make it available to more people? Is that a concept that would be totally ridiculous, or is that one that you would be willing to maybe explore?

Mr. HAWKINS. I don't think it is ridiculous at all, Mr. Chairman. The same day that the CEO of GM came out and made that statement about the sheer cost of health care there was an article in the Wall Street Journal, and I will be happy to get you a copy of it for the record. A company named Quad Graphics in Wisconsin, it is a printing company, and it does business with Mars Bars and M&M and places all over the country. It makes the wrapper paper. The article pointed out that Quad Graphics is a relatively small employer. It has got printing plants around the country. It was fed up with its increasing health insurance costs, and it opened up a primary care center in its main printing plant in Wisconsin and watched its total health care bill drop like a rock.

Mr. WHITFIELD. Really?

Mr. HAWKINS. Yes. Saving 15 percent or more in health care spending. They are, obviously, a self-insured plan. So they reap the benefits of the investment in that primary care center. It is a measure for the ages, because it is not just any kind of primary care when you have organized primary care with a focus on, through the collaboratives, providing quality care, the kind of standards that health centers must operate under. And then I would argue, the strong community oversight that ensures that that center responds to the real local problems, that is the measure for success.

Mr. WHITFIELD. Right.

Mr. HAWKINS. And I think that Quad Graphics got it right, as one business.

Mr. WHITFIELD. Would you give us a copy of that?

Mr. HAWKINS. I would be glad to do so, sir.

Mr. WHITFIELD. All right. Provide that for us.

Do you have any questions, Mr. Stupak?

Mr. STUPAK. Mr. Chairman, I want to ask Ms. Sibilsky this.

You all do a great job, and I am seeing this. I am really concerned about this expansion on community health centers and how we are going to get reimbursed. It just seems to me, and I tried to get more out of Mr. Smith that during these difficult economic times, while Michigan is having it, and I am sure other parts of the country are, too, that Medicare reimbursement should be going up as you are seeing more and more people. And I think I pointed to Michigan with a 30-percent increase but yet we have been able to hold the cost at about 5 percent.

Ms. SIBILSKY. Right.

Mr. STUPAK. And when I was trying to ask these questions, I kept hearing about other sources of funding and all of that. And the only other sources of funding that I really know or see is your great job in getting private contributions into the system. And it certainly helps out a lot. And you mentioned this in your written testimony about the prospective payment system gives community health centers a higher fee per office visit than a private physician would receive, and you explained that at a center might include other services not included in an office visit with a private doctor. Could you explain that a little bit more just to clarify it for me?

Ms. SIBILSKY. Right. An encounter is the terminology we use, and an encounter is all of the services delivered to an individual in a day at a health center for medical. Now since we have gone into mental health and substance abuse services and dental care, you could actually have three encounters a day. But if you are talking about the medical encounter, it can include lab, it can include x-ray, it can include education, our whole bundle, pharmacy. It is the whole bundle of services delivered to an individual in 1 day is one encounter.

Mr. STUPAK. So the reimbursement is for that one encounter?

Ms. SIBILSKY. Correct.

Mr. STUPAK. Okay. So if I go in and I have got a bad knee and I want you to look at it, but you might talk to me about——

Ms. SIBILSKY. Your weight.

Mr. STUPAK. What is wrong with it?

Ms. SIBILSKY. Excuse me. I am sorry. I have no intention of——

Mr. STUPAK. I am only teasing. I am only teasing.

Ms. SIBILSKY. I am sorry, Mr. Stupak.

Mr. STUPAK. No, no, no. I am only teasing.

Ms. SIBILSKY. But one person's weight.

Mr. STUPAK. How about my blood pressure being here in Congress?

Ms. SIBILSKY. Okay. Blood pressure.

Mr. STUPAK. So that is the difference. So if I went to a doctor's office, I would get multiple bills, then, would I not, for the service, but not for the encounter of the day?

Ms. SIBILSKY. Yes, you would. Absolutely.

Mr. STUPAK. I see. I see.

Ms. SIBILSKY. Absolutely. And so when we were talking about it is the benefit of prospective payment to our health centers allowing us to be able to budget, we know, on a prospective basis, what we are going to be receiving from Medicaid.

Mr. STUPAK. Okay.

Ms. SIBILSKY. And so we can project what we can spend.

Mr. STUPAK. Sure.

Ms. SIBILSKY. And it forces us to economize and to creative, in the legal sense of the term, work.

Mr. STUPAK. Okay. But then in your testimony you also talked about how the waiver program may threaten the prospective payment system.

Ms. SIBILSKY. Yes.

Mr. STUPAK. Okay. Explain that.

Ms. SIBILSKY. Well, for example, with the SCHIP program, when it came into Michigan, we were very supportive of that program, of course. And we are not concerned especially about receiving the FQHC prospective payment assurances under SCHIP, because it was going to be for kids.

Mr. STUPAK. Right.

Ms. SIBILSKY. And kids are lower cost. However, under the Michigan adults benefit waiver, as you recall, that is an SCHIP waiver that covers childless adults up to 35 percent of poverty. These are people who have been out of health care, except perhaps through a voucher, for years. And so what it does is it gives the SCHIP payment for adults who are terribly complicated. I mean, Dr. Goetcheus sees these people. They are on the streets. They are dual diagnosis: mental health and substance abuse, and they are expensive. So waiver programs, we believe that population should be served, and we are seeing half to two-thirds of those folks within our clinics, but actually at about 85 percent of fee for service, which is, itself, at about 60 percent of reasonable cost.

Mr. STUPAK. Well, but 60 percent. What are you actually getting paid, then, for these adults? Because SCHIP, it is not very large reimbursement at all.

Ms. SIBILSKY. No, it is probably between $25 and $30 for an encounter.

Mr. STUPAK. For everything for that day?

Ms. SIBILSKY. For everything, because all of the people who we serve receive the same types of services, the FQHC bundle of services.

Mr. STUPAK. And obviously the sliding scale doesn't help you, because there is nothing there.

Ms. SIBILSKY. Thirty-five percent of poverty is about $260 a month.

Mr. HAWKINS. In Medicaid or SCHIP, you can't bill for any underpayment. That would be balance billing. It would violate the Federal statute.

Ms. SIBILSKY. Right.

Mr. STUPAK. Okay.

Mr. WHITFIELD. Dr. Goetcheus, one question I just want to ask you.

You mentioned something about 2,400 individuals are coming from prison back to DC. Is that per year?

Ms. GOETCHEUS. Per year.

Mr. WHITFIELD. Is that right?

Ms. GOETCHEUS. And they are scattered all over the United States.

Mr. WHITFIELD. Each year.

Ms. GOETCHEUS. For instance, in Rivers, North Carolina, there are 1,000 District residents in that prison. What we have set up is some telecommunication so we can try to have, even in groups and individuals, to try to talk with them about when you get back into the District, you need your medications. This is where you come. If you are coming to a homeless shelter, because a lot of them end up in homeless shelters, this is the shelter we want you to come to, because we have a health service there and we want you to come in. And we have social workers there, and we will try to get you jobs. And but it is 2,400 a year coming from the prisons around the United States back into the District and 50 a day coming out of DC jail back into the community.

Mr. WHITFIELD. Per day?

Ms. GOETCHEUS. Per day.

Mr. STUPAK. I found this statement intriguing and the theory. Mr. Hawkins, I think you mentioned it. For 1 percent, you are providing for 10 percent of the people, right?

Mr. HAWKINS. That is correct, Mr. Stupak.

Mr. STUPAK. So in theory, if we gave you 2 percent, could you provide for 20 percent?

Mr. HAWKINS. In theory, yes.

Mr. STUPAK. Could you go 10 percent at 100 percent?

Mr. HAWKINS. For 100 percent?

Mr. STUPAK. No, no, no, 10 percent for 100 percent.

Mr. HAWKINS. Well, and keep in mind, please, that that is 2 percent of total Medicaid spending, which includes hospital and nursing homes.

Mr. STUPAK. Sure.

Mr. HAWKINS. But about 25 percent of Medicaid goes for physician services. And so by dint of that, your math is good. For 10 percent of Medicaid spending, or about half of what is spent on physician services today, yes, we could provide the care for 100 percent of Medicaid beneficiaries. Certainly, for the 40 million who are non-disabled, non-aged. You know, we do have health centers that provide care to frail elderly and disabled individuals, but those who need to be institutionalized in a nursing home or what have you, you know, we do the visits, inpatient visits. I don't know that we could do the long-term care. That is a huge expense. But for the 40 million Medicaid beneficiaries who are adults, children mostly, and relatively non-disabled adults, yes, we could do it. And we would save, just as we do now, Medicaid more money today than all of the money that Medicaid pays health centers. In effect, they get that care for free, and we still give them a further return on investment. The savings exceed the $2.5 billion that Medicaid pays health centers today compared to any other providers. That is what the record shows. So for 10 percent of the dollars, we would give you 100 percent of the patients and give you an even greater return. Lower hospitalizations, fewer specialty referrals, most importantly, a healthier population.

Mr. STUPAK. Sure. Someone said, you know, that they feel that health care is a right and not necessarily a privilege in this country. If we did the uninsured population and gave them the option, if you will, of moving either into a CHIPs program, a Medicare program, or a Federal health employees benefit package, in your opinion, would it be—I am trying to find a way to ensure, you know, everyone who doesn't have health care coverage, and we are actually working on some legislation to do this, to give them an option. If you are child is on the SCHIP program, or in Michigan we call it "My Child", why can't that, usually a single parent, get on the program, too? Or going through the Medicaid program, why can't people under 65 buy into the Medicare system sooner? Why can't those who fall in between come into the Federal employees' health benefit package, because I am sure you must see Federal employees at some of your clinics, because we are in remote areas? I am just trying to find a way to find coverage and at the same time keep the costs reasonable for everybody. Comments on that crazy utopian idea?

Mr. HAWKINS. No, no, not necessarily.

I think two things, too. I mean, the question you want to ask is for the 6 counties in your District and for the 16 in yours, Mr. Chairman, that don't have a health center today and our poor county. Their low-income population is above the national average. Why can't they have a health center? You asked that earlier of the appropriate authorities.

Mr. STUPAK. Right.

Mr. HAWKINS. I wish I could answer it. If only we had it. I think in an ideal world, something like that, giving people a choice but giving them an option of coverage, would be incredibly important.

I just want to say one other thing. I am no Ellen Greenspan, but I think there is a business argument to be made for the fact that we are not competitive in this global environment, because of the costly fragmented health care system we have today with multiple payers, each of whom plays games and tries to push the cost off on somebody else.

Mr. STUPAK. Sure.

Mr. HAWKINS. I think there is a good business argument to be made for a system, and I don't understand why America's businesses, GM included, they are the first ones to be speaking out. They are picking up 50 percent of the tab today. I don't understand why they are not demanding change for this. But I am not in that part of the business world.

Mr. STUPAK. Thank you, Mr. Chairman.

Mr. WHITFIELD. Thank you.

I just want to ask one brief question, and then we will conclude.

On this issue of physicians, we touched on it a little bit, but how difficult is it to find physicians, and what are the retention issues? And would you all comment on that, those of you involved?

Mr. MANIFOLD. I will make a comment on that.

We have had awfully good luck at Central Virginia over the years. Now one of the reasons why we have that luck, and it is not luck in that sense, is because of the support systems, for example the National Health Service Corps has helped us to recruit. But we have also had good relationships with the two teaching institutions in Virginia, the Medical College of Virginia and the University of Virginia. And with those arrangements, we actually, in our particular situation, and I know there are other health centers that do this, we actually teach residents at our site. Medical residents come out. We even have had dental students over the years. And now we have psychology students coming out to our sites and being taught. And that helps us to get to know them. They get to know us. Those kind of arrangements like that, where we have a good teaching kind of relationship, does help us to find good providers along the way, and we have even had people who said, "Gosh, I came out here to your health center. I learned something. I don't want to be a primary care doctor. I am going into surgery." You know. "This is not what I want to do."

Mr. WHITFIELD. Right.

Mr. MANIFOLD. So you have both sides of that coin, and that is a good thing, because had that gentleman come to us at work and then said, "Wait a minute here. I don't like this," the connection with the teaching institution is very strong.

Mr. WHITFIELD. Ms. Sibilsky?

Ms. SIBILSKY. Yes, I would like to support what Mr. Manifold said. I would also like to cite an example of that where 100 percent of the fourth year dental students at the University of Michigan are rotating through community health centers, and as a result, the recruitment rates have just escalated beautifully because they have learned that they are valued organizations and in good communities. Also, the Area Health Education Center, the AHEC program, funded to the Bureau of Health Professions, which we were just funded for in Michigan about a year ago, is starting to develop those kinds of relationships for us. Also, the waiver program has been a real benefit. And we have found amazing acceptability of those providers within rural and remote communities. So thank you.

Mr. SHI. I just want to add that in addition to physicians, nonphysician primary care providers also are the backbone in community health centers. Those include nurse practitioners, physician assistants, and other advanced nurses. And we did studies showing that they provided comparable quality care to primary care physicians in most of the primary care services.

Mr. WHITFIELD. Right. Good point. Good point.

Dr. Goetcheus?

Ms. GOETCHEUS. I would just echo the same. We have relationships with all of the medical schools. There are three here in DC that have students and residents, have four family practice fellows that spend clinical time with us has been a wonderful way to recruit, but the most important way has been because of National

Health Corps. And one of the things I always say is that because many of the physicians who have come to us are minority. And some of them have grown up in these very neighborhoods where they have been out east of the river, and what a wonderful witness that is to that community. So I don't know, we could not, in terms of recruitment, do it. It would be much more difficult without National Health Corps. I am just, every day, grateful for it.

Mr. HAWKINS. I would just say nationally that one thing health centers have learned over the last 40 years is there are three strategies to recruit and keep your staff. No. 1, get your staff involved with teaching hospitals. They are part of that system. They are not renegades and mavericks and lone rangers. They are actually mainstream. No. 2, expose those new, soon-to-be doctors to the experience of working in a health center, and you will, more often than not, have someone who is very interested in coming to work for you down the line. And the third successful strategy that many health centers have employed is grow your own. Find young people in your community who have the promise and the hope and who look like the people you serve and help send them off to get an education, a medical education, a dental education, a nursing education, and they will come back. They will come back and serve the community that grew them.

Ms. SIBILSKY. I would like to give Mr. Stupak an example of that. I was the administrator of the health center in Alcona County, which is one of yours, and I think this was about 20 years ago. I was administering that clinic, and a young medical student came in, and he said to me, "Do you think you will be recruiting doctors in about 10 years when I come out of medical school and residency program?" I said, "I venture to say we would be delighted to have you, and I would almost give you a guarantee of hire." He came back in 10 years and was also married to a doctor, and we got two out of that one.

Mr. STUPAK. That is great. You know, you mentioned doctors, but what about nurses? One of the questions I was going to ask earlier, you know, we had the nurse reinvestment act on this committee, and I think we all supported it. And back last time we had a nurse shortage I think was in the mid 1970's or so. Back then, Congress put in like $150 million to help nurses, to recruit them and pay for their education. Well, I think it was actually $153 million. This past year, we only put in $150 million. I mean, in 30 years, if my math is right, we haven't increased the funding for the program, but yet the demand is just as great. I mean, in the 1970's, we had it for a while and then it went away. Now it is back again, because we have this shortage. Do you recruit and use nurses? And you must, in your fields all of the time, right?

Ms. GOETCHEUS. It is one of our most difficult people to recruit is to get nurses. It is very, very difficult. And as we are talking about the collaboratives and the importance of education and care management, the nurses are key here. And so at least for us, it has been very, very difficult to recruit nurses.

Mr. STUPAK. And the nurses we talked to, they say at $150 million, which was 30 years ago, like 98 percent of them are rejected for any financial aid, even though we have this great need for nurses. I mean, I just can't figure this one out other than we need some more bucks here just to help them out. I mean, they are not asking for a lot, just a little help with their schooling and come work in your clinics and centers. It would be of great help to us all.

Mr. HAWKINS. Health centers are up against shortages in any number of areas. Nursing is one. Dentists. The number of dentists are declining in the dental school. We actually started, we, the National Association, working with a medical school to help start a dental school, because the need is so great. Primary care physicians, pharmacists, and mental health counselors are all in significantly short supply.

Mr. STUPAK. Thank you.

Mr. MANIFOLD. We have six dental sites in our Central Virginia family, and four of the positions are filled right now and two are not filled. And we have a mighty strong effort. We have gotten some changes to Virginia law that helps to allow for more dentists to come into the State. And it is still virtually a nightmare for us, because we have the money, we have the chairs, we have everything we need, and it is still very, very difficult to find those dentists.

Mr. WHITFIELD. Well, I want to thank you all so much for your testimony. We really enjoyed spending Wednesday afternoon with you, and I am sure Mr. Stupak and I both would say that we look forward to maintaining contact with you as we move forward to try to address some of these issues. So thank you for your time and your testimony.

And I will say that we will keep the record open for 30 days, and we are going to ask members to submit any questions that they have for the record within the next 7 days.

And with that, the hearing is adjourned.

[Whereupon, at 6:03 p.m., the subcommittee was adjourned.]

[Additional material submitted for the record follows:]

DOCUMENTS FOR THE RECORD

1. "States Rein in Health Costs; Legislatures are Looking to Cut Medicaid or Add Fees," *The Los Angeles Times*, April 24, 2005.

2. "Needy Patients Find Door Shut When Looking for Specialist," *The Chicago Tribune*, May 15, 2005.

3. "Cardiology, With Heart," *The Washington Post,* May 24, 2005.

4. "The Reinstatement of Oral Health Benefits for Medicaid Adults: A Defining Moment," Michigan Primary Care Association, undated.

5. "Inequality in America: The Contribution of Health Centers in Reducing and Eliminating Disparities in Access to Care," *Medical Care Research and Review*, June 2001, pp. 234-48.

6. "2004 National Healthcare Disparities Report," Agency for Healthcare Research and Quality.

7. "Medicaid Programs Enticing to States with Budget Problems," *Lab Business Week*, Feb. 27, 2005

8. "Medicaid Acute Care Services," *The Medicaid Resource Book,* Kaiser Commission on Medicaid and the Uninsured, July 2002

LexisNexis

Los Angeles Times

April 24, 2005 Sunday
Home Edition

SECTION: MAIN NEWS; National Desk; Part A; Pg. 1

LENGTH: 1940 words

HEADLINE: States Rein In Health Costs;
Legislatures are looking to cut **Medicaid** or add fees. Missouri is poised to end the program, which many of the poor rely upon for care.

BYLINE: Stephanie Simon, Times Staff Writer

DATELINE: SIKESTON, Mo.

BODY:

Hundreds of thousands of poor people across the nation will lose their state-subsidized health insurance in the coming months as legislators scramble to hold down the enormous -- and ever-escalating -- cost of **Medicaid.**

Here in impoverished southeast Missouri, nurses at a family health clinic stash drug samples for patients they know won't be able to afford their prescriptions after their coverage is eliminated this summer. Doctors try to comfort waitresses, sales clerks and others who will soon lose coverage for medical, dental and mental healthcare.

"I don't know what cure to offer them," Dr. Hameed Khaja said.

Lawmakers say they feel for those who will lose coverage. But they say also that they have no alternative.

Prenatal checkups, care in nursing homes and other health services for the poor and disabled account for more than 25% of total spending in many states. **Medicaid** is often a state's single biggest budget item, more expensive even than K-12 education. And the price of services, especially prescription drugs and skilled nursing for the elderly, continues to soar.

The federal government helps pay for **Medicaid,** but in the coming fiscal year, the federal contribution will drop by more than $1 billion because of changes in the cost-share formula. President Bush has warned of far deeper cuts to come; he aims to reduce federal spending on **Medicaid** by as much as $40 billion over the next decade.

"It's frightening a lot of governors," said Diane Rowland, executive director of the Kaiser Commission on **Medicaid** and the Uninsured.

Every state has frozen or is trying to cut the fees they pay doctors to care for **Medicaid** patients. More than a dozen states are looking for ways to cut the number of people covered -- or reduce their benefits. Several are proposing restructuring the entire program.

In Tennessee, Gov. Phil Bredesen plans to end coverage for more than 320,000 adults, many of them elderly. In California, Gov. Arnold Schwarzenegger wants to shift more **Medicaid** recipients into managed care and require some to pay monthly premiums.

Minnesota may stop insuring 27,000 college students and adults without children. Washington state may require senior citizens to pay $3 for each prescription that **Medicaid** used to provide for free.

South Carolina Gov. Mark Sanford and Florida Gov. Jeb Bush have proposed privatizing **Medicaid.** Bush wants to give recipients vouchers so they can shop around for their own insurance plans. Sanford wants to set up **Medicaid** bank accounts; the state would deposit a fixed sum of money for each patient to spend on medical expenses.

In Missouri, where nearly one in five residents is enrolled in **Medicaid,** Gov. Matt Blunt is poised to sign the most drastic overhaul of all: a bill that would eliminate the program entirely in three years.

Blunt expects that by then, the state will have established an alternative mechanism for helping the poorest of the poor. But the legislation on his desk does not insist on it. It only states that Missouri **Medicaid** will cease on June 30, 2008.

In the meantime, the bill severely cuts the existing program, ending coverage for an estimated 65,000 to 100,000 people.

Legislators are still working out eligibility details. But under one leading proposal a single mother of two who earns $3,800 a year would be considered too wealthy to qualify for Missouri **Medicaid.** The woman's children would still be eligible for free healthcare. But if she gets a better job and starts earning $23,000 a year, they, too, would be bumped off **Medicaid** -- unless she's willing to pay as much as 5% of her income in monthly premiums. The state expects many parents at that income level would be unable or unwilling to pay the premiums, forcing about 24,000 children off the **Medicaid** rolls.

Children who remain on **Medicaid** would continue to receive full benefits, but under legislation expected to take effect this summer, most adults would get a bare-bones package. The program would no longer pay for their dental care, hearing aids, eyeglasses, wheelchairs, hospital beds or even bedpans.

State Rep. Trent Skaggs, a Democrat from Kansas City, considers the new rules cruel, especially at a time when more than 45 million Americans lack insurance. He worries parents will stop working so their income will drop low enough to qualify their family for free care.

Rather than raise costs for minimum-wage clerks, Skaggs suggests increasing insurance premiums for lawmakers who get health coverage through the state. He recently introduced a measure that would have cost the average politician $115 a month -- the measure failed on a close vote.

"That made a complete mockery of the idea that leaders sacrifice first," Skaggs said. "Times are tough, but not so tough that we have to sacrifice?"

The Republican lawmakers who have been leading the **Medicaid** overhaul drive say such criticism distorts their goals.

The cuts are not just about balancing this year's budget, they say. They're about steering **Medicaid** back to its original purpose: to serve as safety net for citizens who are too young, too old, or too ill to help themselves. Turning **Medicaid** into a welfare program for poor but able-bodied adults risks jacking up the costs so high, they say, that the entire system could go bust -- stranding those who most desperately need the state's help.

The cost of Missouri **Medicaid** has doubled in the last six years, to $5 billion. It eats up more than 30% of the state budget. More than 1 million people are enrolled.

"Government is not here to do everything for everybody," said state Rep. Jodi Stefanick, a Republican representing suburban St. Louis. "We have to draw the line somewhere."

Medicaid was enacted in 1965 as a joint federal-state program to provide basic care for poor children, pregnant women and people with disabilities. States administer the program and pay 20% to 50% of the total costs. The federal government funds the remainder. (The federal contribution varies from state to state, with the poorest states receiving the largest amounts.)

States can opt out of **Medicaid,** but since 1982 every state has participated. By law, they must offer specific benefit packages to certain groups, including poor pregnant women and young children. They are also free to go beyond those minimum standards.

Historically, lawmakers have considered it a bargain to go beyond because the federal government pays for so much of the program. So states from California to Maine have expanded **Medicaid** to cover working parents, lower-middle-class children and elderly citizens struggling to pay for the many services not funded by **Medicare.**

The result: **Medicaid** now covers 53 million Americans. The program pays the bills for nearly 60% of all nursing home residents and finances 37% of all births. Because most states have added prescription drug benefits, **Medicaid** covers the hefty pharmacy bills for many patients with AIDS, many transplant recipients and many senior citizens on dialysis or undergoing chemotherapy.

The program also covers the more mundane medical expenses of low-income working families.

Here in Sikeston, Dianna Dixon, 18, relies on **Medicaid** because her 30-hour-a-week job at Wal-Mart does not come with insurance. Her mother, Donna Sevic, uses **Medicaid,** too, now that arthritis has forced her to stop working after years in low-wage restaurant, sales and factory jobs.

Waiting in the Southern Missouri Health Network's clinic the other day to ask a doctor about Dixon's headaches, the women said they expected to lose their coverage this summer. Sevic, 50, said the loss would be devastating; she wasn't sure how she would afford her medications, much less any doctor visits.

"If they take it away from me, I'll just go downhill," Sevic said. "I won't be here much longer. It's that plain and simple." Eyes weary, she said she thought she deserved better: "If you get out and try, really try to make a living, the government ought to step in and help you."

That philosophy still resonates in some states.

In Kansas, Gov. Kathleen Sebelius has proposed raising cigarette taxes to pay for expanding **Medicaid** to cover more poor working adults.

In Illinois, an expansion is underway. In the last two years, Gov. Rod Blagojevich has added tens of thousands of children to the **Medicaid** rolls -- and tens of thousands of parents, as well. "I can't think of anything more important to do," he said.

"Healthy families are working families," added Barry Maram, director of the Illinois Department of Public Aid. "This makes all the economic sense in the world."

The Republicans who dominate the state Legislature in neighboring Missouri offer a different definition of economic sense.

"We're careening out of control," said state Sen. Michael Gibbons, who represents suburban St. Louis. "Taxpayers are not an endless supply of money."

The cutbacks that Gibbons helped craft will save the state $250 million next fiscal year.

They may also cost 73-year-old Mary Bostic her dream of eating something other than soup for supper.

Bostic, a retired garment-factory worker, has been coming to the clinic in Sikeston for months. In the olive-drab dental exam rooms, Dr. Gail Redman has extracted the crumbling stumps of her rotting teeth, one by one.

Bostic's new top denture plate should be arriving soon. She was expecting to get a bottom plate as well. "I was looking forward to a solid meal," she said.

But the clinic is booked solid for the next six months; there's no time to get her the bottom denture before her **Medicaid** coverage runs out. Without the insurance, Bostic can't even contemplate paying for a bottom plate; it would cost her $375 at the clinic's discount rate.

She has trouble understanding why she's in this fix.

"I've worked all my life," Bostic said. "I've paid my taxes. And now, when I get down and out, they don't want to help me."

The clinic's hygienists are starting to call other patients who have been waiting for dentures, to break the news. Their list runs seven pages long.

"It breaks your heart," Redman said, in tears. "They've been waiting so long to get teeth."

In appropriations conferences this week, Missouri legislators could restore some dental care or other benefits to the **Medicaid** package. They may also ease up slightly on the eligibility restrictions. But given the state's budget constraints -- and the majority party's philosophical stance on **Medicaid** -- analysts don't expect a substantial retreat.

That's as it should be, lawmaker Stefanick said. "Once you put a benefit out there, reining it in is not easy," she said. "But it is the responsible thing to do."

*

Major expense

For most states, **Medicaid** expenses are often the single largest line item on the budget, exceeding K-12 education. States spending the most on **Medicaid** as a percentage of fiscal 2004 budgets:

Tennessee... 33.3%

Missouri ...30.7

Pennsylvania ...29.5

Maine ...29.0

New York ...28.3

Illinois... 28.1

Vermont ...27.5

New Hampshire... 26.4

Mississippi... 26.3

Rhode Island ...25.5

Who receives **Medicaid**

* 25 million children

* 13 million low-income adults, including pregnant women

* 15 million seniors and people with disabilities

Medicaid benefits

By federal law, states must provide certain benefits for **Medicaid** recipients, including:

* Inpatient and outpatient hospital services

* Physician, psychiatrist and nurse practitioner visits

* Nursing home and home healthcare for adults

* Family-planning services and supplies

* Lab and X-ray services

* Transportation to medical appointments

Sources: Health Management Associates; National Assn. of State Budget Officers; the Kaiser Commission on **Medicaid** and the Uninsured

Chicago Tribune

May 15, 2005 Sunday
Chicago Final Edition

SECTION: NEWS ; ZONE C; Pg. 1

LENGTH: 2091 words

HEADLINE: Needy patients find door shut when searching for specialist

SERIES: UNINSURED IN AMERICA
In the United States, 45 million citizens have no health insurance and their ranks are growing. With this report the Tribune begins an ongoing examination of the uninsured and the problems they face.

BYLINE: By Judith Graham, Tribune staff reporter.

BODY:

Sandra Herron's health was taking a sharp turn for the worse. It was becoming hard to breathe. Lesions were sprouting around her nose. She was tired all the time.

Herron worried it was a serious flare-up of the chronic inflammatory disease she has had for 24 years--a clear signal she needed help from a doctor who specialized in her illness, sarcoidosis.

But Herron, 51, a part-time psychology instructor, didn't have health insurance and couldn't afford to pay a specialist's fees. Not sick enough to go to an emergency room, too distressed to ignore her symptoms, and without a regular doctor to ask for advice, she was at a loss for where to turn.

Millions of uninsured Americans face a similar challenge. Although basic medical services for the needy are available at community clinics across the country, specialty care is scarce for people without health insurance.

"It's the biggest hole in the safety net," said Patricia Terrell, the former deputy chief of Cook County's Bureau of Health Services.

Several factors are fueling a growing sense of crisis surrounding specialty care for the uninsured. The number of people without medical coverage, now estimated at 45 million, is rising steadily, and experts project the trend will continue.

As a group, the uninsured tend to have more chronic illnesses than the population at large. Medical complications requiring specialists' attention also are more common because these patients often forgo routine medical care.

At the same time, public hospitals, which provide the bulk of care to the uninsured, are under intense financial pressure as governments cut back support. Though physicians and private hospitals offer some free or discounted services, they are not sufficient to meet demand.

The result is that uninsured patients with conditions ranging from diabetes to arthritis to Parkinson's disease don't get regular consultations with the doctors who know best how to treat their conditions.

The health consequences are dire: "People get sicker, they die earlier, or they end up with disabling conditions that can create problems throughout the remainder of their lives," said Diane Rowland, executive director of the Kaiser Commission on Medicaid and the Uninsured.

Cancer is an example. Every year, 200,000 uninsured cancer patients spend more than twice as much out of pocket on medical services even though they see doctors far less often than patients with insurance, according to research by experts at Emory University's school of public health.

People with insurance also get sophisticated medical tests such as MRI scans, high-tech services such as heart bypass operations, and preventive screenings such as colonoscopies at much higher rates than those without.

"It's time to examine the current state of specialty care for the uninsured in our communities and talk seriously about what health-care systems across the area can and should be doing," said Donna Thompson, chief executive of Access Community Health Network, which runs 44 clinics for the medically underserved.

New research confirms the scope of the problem. Marsha Regenstein, professor of health policy at George Washington University, recently completed a survey of public hospital systems in 10 cities, including Boston and Detroit. In every case, access to specialty services was limited, poorly coordinated with primary care or extremely confusing to patients.

"This is a crisis of national proportions," Regenstein said.

Payment upfront--in cash

American medicine is flush with specialists, experts who know particular body systems or diseases inside-out and stay on top of the most advanced treatments. For someone with insurance, access to these physicians is usually as easy as calling for an appointment.

But if a patient without insurance contacts a private doctor's office, he will typically be asked for payment upfront--in cash. If he doesn't have the money, he often is politely asked to seek care elsewhere.

"There are very few physicians in private practice who make themselves available to the uninsured," said Alan Channing, chief executive officer of Sinai Health System in Chicago, where one out of every five patients has no medical coverage.

If a patient tries a community clinic for the medically needy, and a doctor there finds a problem that needs a more expert examination--let's say, a suspicious mass in the abdomen--the options are limited.

Often, "the doctor will pick up the phone and call a specialist he knows, asking for a favor: Please, can you see this patient; she really needs attention," said Bruce Johnson, executive director of the Illinois Primary Health Care Association. Specialists will frequently agree to help a colleague.

If that doesn't work, patients often seek specialty care at hospital emergency rooms. But that isn't a good solution for the 1.8 million Illinoisans without medical coverage.

Though hospitals are required to treat patients in medical crises, there's no such requirement for non-emergency or follow-up care--the kind of specialty services that are most needed and hardest to get.

Most community hospitals supply only limited amounts of charity care, and then mostly for patients with acute conditions. As a rule, their specialists are in private practice and don't take many patients without insurance.

There are exceptions: Some private institutions, such as Mt. Sinai Hospital and St. Anthony's Hospital in Chicago, among others, open their doors to large numbers of indigent patients.

Academic medical centers once offered a fairly substantial amount of care. But now, under financial pressure, specialists at these institutions are treating more people with private insurance and fewer of the uninsured.

A 2003 study by researchers at Boston's Massachusetts General Hospital documents the trend: Of 2,000 physicians surveyed across the country, one in four said they had problems admitting uninsured patients to teaching hospitals or were forced to limit those patients' care

Public institutions like Stroger Hospital are the largest providers of specialized medical services to the uninsured. Patients who get basic medical care from these hospitals' clinics also are eligible for more advanced care.

But getting an appointment can take months. And patients who try to see a specialist without a referral from an affiliated doctor won't get to see one.

"At most public hospitals, the attitude has been, `We'll do a great job for you as long as you can get in the door.' But good luck getting in," said Dr. Terry Conway, an internist who splits his time between Cook County's sprawling health-care system and a consulting practice.

`I get so worried'

On a recent rainy morning, Sandra Herron was wondering how she was going to do it all--get expensive tests, arrange for specialty care, pay for needed medicines--as she sat in the crowded waiting room of an Access Community Health clinic in Chicago Heights.

A part-time social worker and psychology instructor at South Suburban College, Herron has known for 24 years that she has sarcoidosis, an inflammatory disease that can cause lumps to form in the lungs and other organs.

Most of the time, her symptoms were manageable, and she thought she could get by without medical checkups or insurance, which she dropped about five years ago because of the expense.

That changed in January after she started waking up gasping for air in the middle of the night and her son took her to the emergency room at South Suburban Hospital in Hazel Crest.

Three months and several doctor visits later--but still without a specialist managing her condition--she was having trouble breathing on a regular basis, nasty-looking bumps were popping up around her nostrils, and she was scared.

"I get so worried that I don't know what's going on with my body, and that I'm getting worse," Herron said.

On this dismal spring day, she decided to go to a federally funded health clinic for the medically needy in search of help, and it was Dr. Kevin Gordon's turn to take a look at her.

"This is really not something I know much about," he said after an examination. Gordon, a family physician, proposed referring her to a pulmonologist at Mt. Sinai Hospital.

"That's an hour from where I live: I want something closer to home in case I have another attack," Herron responded.

Doctor and patient agreed her best strategy was to go to Oak Forest Hospital, part of Cook County's sprawling health system, and try to get a referral from an emergency room physician to a pulmonologist.

It would be a long wait, but it was also her best bet, Gordon told Herron, who later acknowledged she was nervous about what lay ahead.

What would the hospital bill her for the services? How could she pay for further treatments with other unpaid medical bills sitting at home? And what if something were to happen to her before she saw a specialist and she again suffered that devastating feeling of not getting enough air into her lungs?

"If only clinics like these had it so those who cannot afford much could still go to a specialist around where they live, it wouldn't be nearly so scary," Herron sighed.

If Herron's medical concerns had been the kind general doctors see every day--say, an infection--she wouldn't have had to worry so much.

Over the last decade, the federal government has poured significant amounts of money into expanding neighborhood health clinics for the needy, increasing the capacity to deliver basic care. Boosting the number of such centers is a significant priority for the Bush administration.

In Illinois, 43 federally qualified health centers now offer services at 250 sites across the state to 850,000 patients--including 325,000 without insurance--every year, according to the Illinois Primary Health Care Association.

Yet the federal government hasn't devoted funding to expanding specialty care; neither have most local and state governments.

Without a reliable funding stream, "these [specialty] services just aren't readily available," said Conway, who consults widely with public hospital systems across the country.

Specialists in short supply

Aggravating the situation is a nationwide shortage of certain specialists--for instance, orthopedists and radiologists.

Few choose to practice in disadvantaged locations, with demand for their services high, and with much more money to be made in the suburbs.

"Even if we had lots and lots of extra money, we still couldn't totally staff our clinics," said Dr. Daniel Winship, chief of Cook County's Bureau of Health Services, which runs three hospitals and 28 clinics across the city and suburbs.

Oak Forest Hospital, for example, lost its sole gastroenterologist--a doctor that handles diseases of the digestive system--last year and has not yet been able to replace him. As a result, patients from the south suburbs have to find their way to Stroger Hospital, where waits in the gastroenterology clinic now extend about 12 months, Winship said.

The chaos surrounding specialty care plays out every day in Chicago Heights at Access Family Health Society, the center run by Access Community Health, the nation's largest chain of federally funded clinics for the needy.

On a recent morning, Gordon paused between exams to describe the difficulties he routinely faces when a sick patient walks in the door.

"If the person doesn't have insurance, I can't order up MRI or CT scans even if I think they're necessary," he said. "The best I can do, usually, is to send them over to the Oak Forest Hospital emergency room and hope they can get it done over there."

Once a patient goes off to the hospital, however, "I don't have much control over what happens," Gordon said. "Often, you lose them and just hope everything turned out all right."

"Sometimes I'm on the phone for hours at a time, trying to make things work," chimed in Dr. Cynthia Thomas, the clinic's medical director.

Although the Chicago Heights clinic has a referral relationship with specialists at Mt. Sinai Hospital, many south suburban patients don't have a way to get to the West Side hospital. Others can't afford even the scaled-back fees that Sinai physicians charge patients without insurance.

Thomas remembered a patient the week before with kidney stones who needed to see a urologist and get two important diagnostic tests. After negotiating reduced rates at Mt. Sinai through a financial counselor, Thomas told the woman what she'd pay: at least $50 for the urologist, $70 for the ultrasound, $100 for the CT scan.

It was a fraction of the true cost, but it was too much.

"She just started crying," Thomas said.

jegraham@tribune.com

GRAPHIC: PHOTO: Dr. Kevin Gordon talks with medical assistant Ruelena Castillo at a Chicago Heights clinic that serves the needy. Uninsured patients pose challenges, he says. "If the person doesn't have insurance, I can't order up MRI or CT scans even if I think they're necessary." Tribune photos by John Smierciak.

PHOTO: Sandra Herron, whose chronic illness has worsened, is unsure how she will arrange for specialty care without insurance.
PHOTOS 2

LOAD-DATE: May 15, 2005

The Washington Post
washingtonpost.com
The Washington Post

May 24, 2005 Tuesday
Final Edition

SECTION: Health; F01

LENGTH: 2276 words

HEADLINE: Cardiology, With Heart;
Most Poor, Under-Insured Patients Don't Get Adequate Care From Specialists. One Doctor Is Doing What She Can to Meet the Need.

BYLINE: Sandra G. Boodman, Washington Post Staff Writer

BODY:

"This is a mess," cardiologist Nancy J. Davenport declares as she examines the hugely swollen legs of Jerone Browner-El, who sits slumped on a stool in an office at Washington Hospital Center looking miserable and angry.

"You're like the popping fresh doughboy, baby," Davenport adds gently, scanning the list of medicines the 56-year-old Northeast Washington resident is supposed to be taking. The drugs are supposed to control his blood pressure, rein in his diabetes and shore up his badly enlarged heart. Because his kidneys are failing, his feet are so swollen he can barely stuff them into soft shoes that resemble bedroom slippers. His blood pressure is dangerously high.

Davenport zeroes in on that first, asking Browner-El whether he is taking the hypertension medicines she gave him. Sometimes, he replies, scowling. His wife quickly interjects, assuring Davenport, who has been her doctor for several years, that her husband is mad at her for making him go to the doctor.

"We are a mess," she says to Davenport. "You're the reason, along with God's grace, that I'm here today," she adds. This time, she tells Davenport, it is her husband who needs help.

So do a growing number of low-income Washington area residents who are facing an acute shortage of doctors, particularly specialists, willing to treat them.

In the District, an estimated 15 percent of the population has no health insurance and one in three residents receives health benefits from a patchwork of government programs. Those covered by Medicaid, the government program for the poor and disabled, are increasingly unable to find doctors willing to care for them because of the program's low reimbursement rate. The same problem affects the thousands enrolled in the D.C. Healthcare Alliance, a network of doctors and hospitals launched six years ago, two years before the city's only public hospital, D.C. General, was closed.

"It's really hard for people without adequate health insurance to get cardiovascular care," said Paul Ginsburg, an economist who directs the Center for Studying Health System Change, a nonprofit Washington think tank.

"Doctors who offer pro bono [services] or discounted fees are few and far between," said Carolyn Gardner, director of the Washington Free Clinic. Finding specialists remains a huge challenge for her staff, she said. For patients with heart problems, the clinic relies on the services of a lone cardiologist who comes to the Mount Pleasant clinic once a month. Frequently, she said, her staff has to "get on the phone and beg, borrow and steal" to obtain appointments for patients with other specialists.

Follow-up care is essential for cardiac patients because heart problems tend to be chronic and often occur in conjunction with diabetes, hypertension and lung ailments. Numerous studies have found that people who receive only episodic treatment for these problems tend to suffer from needless disability and premature death.

Because patients often wait months to see a specialist, many wind up in crisis in swamped emergency rooms. Doctors there are required to take care of them during a crisis, but not to provide the continuing care that might prevent a recurrence.

Davenport, one of the Washington area's few female interventional cardiologists -- heart specialists with advanced training who perform angioplasty and other invasive procedures -- is an exception. Although she sees about 100 patients per week in her own office in upper Northwest, two Saturdays a month she holds a **cardiology** clinic for less affluent patients, many of whom who live in medically under-served areas of the District.

Using an office borrowed from another cardiologist and with assistance from medical students from Georgetown, where Davenport teaches, she dispenses advice and encouragement and gives away large quantities of free drug samples in plastic shopping bags she brings from home. She arranges for tests and follow-up care for her growing roster of established patients, as well as a steady stream of new ones, some referred by other doctors or hospitals or their friends or relatives. A minority of patients are homeless; others live as far away as Calvert County.

A few patients arrive without an appointment and are seen anyway. The majority are enrolled in Medicaid or the D.C. Healthcare Alliance, which covers poor people who don't qualify for Medicaid.

Many of the 20 or so patients who typically show up for the Saturday clinic -- taxi drivers, recovering drug addicts, hotel workers, former prisoners and the elderly -- would be unlikely to see a heart specialist outside an emergency room. Most have a serious cardiovascular problem, sometimes several of them. A surprising number are in their forties and have survived at least one major stroke or heart attack.

Unlike most heart specialists, "Nancy has an open-door policy," said Tom Norin, the administrator of her large practice, which follows about 3,000 patients.

While many physicians decry paltry insurance reimbursements and complain they must work harder to compensate for rising malpractice insurance costs, Davenport, who is board-certified in internal medicine, cardiovascular diseases and interventional **cardiology,** shows no interest in the financial aspects of medicine.

"The truth is that she's the least interested of any physician I've ever met in making money," Norin added. "I have to literally chase her down to get her to talk about it."

Norin said the clinic, at which he sometimes volunteers, was started more than a decade ago by a former partner of Davenport's; her new associate Getu Assefa sometimes helps out. Echocardiography technician John Galvin also donates his time on a few Saturdays during the year, performing tests that cost about $600 each on clinic patients.

Davenport, who adores talking about **cardiology,** is much less forthcoming about herself. She looks surprised when asked why she continues to operate a clinic that adds to her prodigious workload. In exchange for borrowing the hospital center office of cardiologist H. Brandis Marsh and dispensing his large stash of samples to her patients, Davenport makes rounds for him every weekend.

"I feel responsible," she says simply. When asked to elaborate, she observes that many clinic patients would be unable or unwilling to travel to her office.

Davenport has a tart sense of humor, boundless energy and a direct, unflappable manner that befits a nurse, which was the first of her three careers. Now 59 and a grandmother, she left a tenured professorship in nursing at American University to enter George Washington University School of Medicine at 35. She'd already earned a doctorate in cardiac physiology at GWU and worked for two years as a postdoctoral fellow in a lab at the National Institutes of Health (NIH).

At the time she entered medical school, Davenport and her husband had four young sons, and her husband was establishing his career as a Washington litigator specializing in complex product liability cases. Their daughter, now 17, was born during Davenport's residency at Georgetown.

Davenport grew up in a medical family: Her mother was a nurse and her father was a prominent Chicago surgeon. She said she decided to go to medical school because she was irked that a physician's signature was required for routine blood draws at NIH. "I decided I wasn't going to be the bottom person on the totem pole," she said.

Her practice is located in the upscale Foxhall Square medical building on New Mexico Avenue NW. She routinely works 90-hour weeks, shuttling among Sibley Hospital, Suburban Hospital and Washington Hospital Center, sometimes staying up until 4 a.m. performing cardiac catheterizations on patients who've had heart attacks.

Davenport displays none of the status consciousness common among high-powered specialists: She tidies up the exam rooms and empties the trash after her clinic is over and recently walked out to the waiting room to apologize to a patient who had been waiting 30 minutes to see her. She doesn't own a cell phone or PDA or use e-mail.

"Nancy is a first-rate person in all respects," said Marsh, the cardiologist whose office she borrows. "She knows her **cardiology,** she pays attention, she follows up and she seems to enjoy the kind of personal relationship with her patients that was the neat thing about medicine when I started. Nancy is never too busy to do something for someone else."

Before she met Davenport in the emergency room of Washington Hospital Center six years ago, Carolyn Browner-El said doctors elsewhere had minimized her complaints of chest pains and sent her home with nitroglycerin.

Davenport, she said, was different. She performed several tests and then did a cardiac catheterization, determining that Browner-El had a weak heart because of cardiomyopathy, a condition that affects the heart's pumping ability. Now 49, she became one of Davenport's patients and her heart problem improved.

"Dr. Davenport gave me a regimen of medicines that stabilized my heart, and now I see her once a year," said Browner-El, who said her family income is about $1,200 per month. She is now struggling with a more serious problem: Her liver is failing and she needs a transplant. But when she and her husband came to the clinic last month, Davenport was more worried about Jerone.

Davenport tells the couple she will call another kidney specialist -- the fourth she has contacted on his behalf -- to ask if he will see Browner-El. She gives him a follow-up appointment, reminds him to take his blood pressure medicine and asks if he needs a coupon for a free home blood pressure cuff.

As she heads for the next patient, one of two pagers clipped to her white coat emits a piercing beep. The emergency room at Georgetown has a 40-year-old woman who may need a cardiac catheterization. Davenport tells Georgetown to send the patient to the hospital center and she'll see the woman after her clinic closes around 2 p.m. -- and before she heads to Suburban Hospital to make rounds there.

Two Saturdays later, Davenport is in the clinic by 9 a.m. Usually her daughter, Gina, serves as the receptionist, but this time it is her husband, Jim, who is wearing jeans, a T-shirt and running shoes.

Robert Dent, the first of the day's 20 patients, arrives 15 minutes early for his appointment. At 56, he has survived a near-fatal heart attack and a less serious one, as well as a blood clot. He has artificial hips and knee replacements, wears a pacemaker and has undergone surgery on his shoulder. Retired on total disability, he takes medicine for high blood pressure, elevated cholesterol, and heart and lung problems.

He met Davenport in 2003, when he was taken by medevac to Washington Hospital Center from Fort Washington Hospital near his home in Prince George's County. She performed angioplasty, but the artery later closed up and last year he had his second heart attack. Davenport performed a second angioplasty, this time combined with low-dose radiation to keep the artery open. So far, it seems to be working, and Dent says he is faithfully taking his medications.

"That's my girl right there," Dent says, grinning broadly as Davenport greets him with her customarily cheery "Hi, sweetie."

Dent, who is dependent on Medicaid, said he particularly appreciates the samples of the seven drugs Davenport gives him. Once he had to pay for them, and he recalled "I couldn't get them all, because they would have eaten up all my [$500] monthly check."

Davenport congratulates her next patient, a 47-year-old former hotel laundry worker, on his normal blood pressure and abstinence from drugs. Davenport met the man a year earlier while he was spending three months in the hospital recovering from a stroke he said was induced by his crack cocaine habit. The man is so pleased about his blood pressure that he asks "Miss Davenport" to write the numbers on a piece of paper so he can show his mother.

She declines to give a D.C. cab driver, who has shown up without an appointment, more Viagra samples along with his other medications because she suspects he may be selling them. "One a day for personal use, okay, but 10? Come on," she says later. "He's not getting any more."

Davenport says that while smoking, drug use, high-fat diets, alcoholism and other bad habits are common among her patients, she doesn't lecture them, believing it would be counterproductive.

But she admits to occasional frustration. A few months ago she had a talk with a patient whose lengthy list of life-threatening medical problems is exacerbated by her morbid obesity. Davenport felt she'd gotten through until she walked by the Blimpie restaurant in the hospital lobby an hour later and spotted the woman tucking into an order of french fries.

Jerone Browner-El is back, looking much more chipper than two weeks earlier. He tells Davenport that the nephrologist she found for him tweaked his medicines in the hope of avoiding dialysis and draining the 30 pounds of fluid that have accumulated in his legs.

Davenport tells him she is glad to see that his blood pressure is lower than last time, and he replies, looking somewhat sheepish, that he is taking his pills.

When the doctor asks about his wife, Browner-El tells Davenport that doctors at another hospital have told Carolyn there is nothing more they can do to treat her failing liver.

"They may not be able to get her a [new] liver, but someone can take care of her," Davenport says. "And if they won't, you give me a call and I'll poll some of my GI [gastroenterology] buddies and see if they'll take her." *

LOAD-DATE: May 24, 2005

The Reinstatement of Oral Health Benefits for Medicaid Adults: *A Defining Moment*

Michigan is at a crossroads. Are we the type of state that makes crucial public policy decisions based on popularity contests that have short-term savings even though they have long-term and far reaching negative outcomes? Or, are we the type of state that engages in thoughtful discussion to determine the most cost-effective manner to do the best for our citizens? Most of us would agree that the Medicaid program is designed to meet both the health care needs of our most vulnerable population in the most cost-effective manner without jeopardizing the financial viability of the provider network in all of Michigan's communities. To achieve these goals, we need to recognize that health is more than primary care physicians and hospitals. We need to appreciate the interplay between oral health, medical care and behavioral health systems.

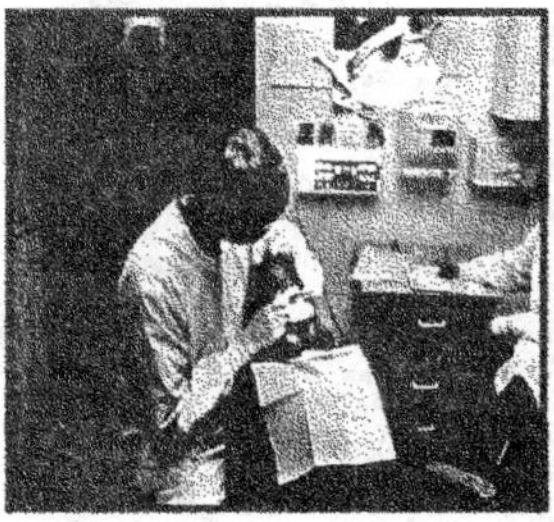

Inattention to oral health has important implications for our ability to reach current and future physical health outcome goals. This has been proven multiple times and published in peer-reviewed journals. Elimination of the Adult Dental Benefit will affect recipients in several ways:

- Pre-term births (before 35 weeks) will increase.
- Diabetes will be more difficult, if not impossible, to control.
- Incidence of arteriosclerosis (narrowing of blood vessels that can lead to a heart attack or stroke) will increase.
- Heart disease will increase.
- Incidence of Low Birth Weight infants will increase.
- Incidence of dental caries in children will increase by inoculation from untreated dental caries in their parents.
- Morbidity and Death from Oral Cancer will increase.
- Untold increase in the incidence and suffering from dental disease.
- Reduced Employability

As clearly demonstrated, dentists are not simply tooth technicians. Dentists are extremely important in preventing, diagnosing and treating both oral and primary health care needs of their patients. The U.S. Surgeon General continues to emphasize the need to eliminate oral disease from the nation's most vulnerable populations in order to preserve their general health. The oral health disparity that exists between the insured and uninsured populations is a national disgrace.

MICHIGAN Primary Care ASSOCIATION

MICHIGAN ASSOCIATION FOR LOCAL PUBLIC HEALTH

Back in 1999, the Michigan State Legislature understood that oral health access is essential if our goals are to improve the health of Medicaid eligibles and limit the exponential growth in Medicaid expenditures. To address the well-documented chronic access problem for the Medicaid population, the state provided $10 million for a three pronged attack. The money was allocated to:

- Provide funds to community clinics, including FQHCs and Local Public Health Departments to establish and expand dental clinics throughout the state,
- Establish Healthy Kids Dental Program in 37 counties, where FQHCs do no exist, which is administered by Delta Dental, and uses Delta's network of participating private practitioners, and
- Provide start-up funds to establish the University of Michigan School of Dentistry Community Outreach Service Learning Program, which allows students to provide care in the community clinic setting.

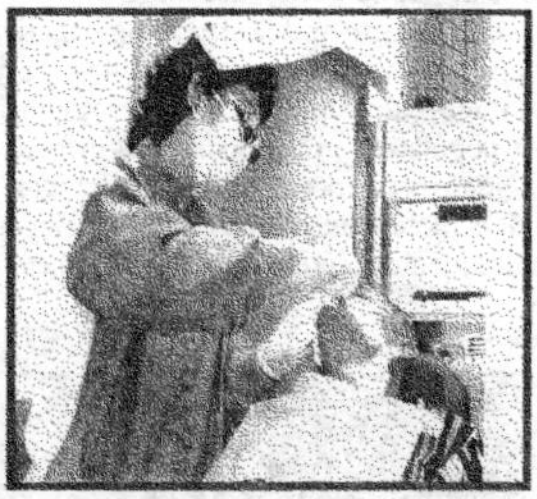

The result of this approach has been an overwhelming success from all three initiatives; and, in just three years since the inception, a significant dent in the unmet need of the Medicaid population has been accomplished. Are we willing to forego this success for only a temporary and relatively small savings?

While eliminating oral health benefits for Medicaid adults will save $9.2 million in up front general fund savings, we believe the actual cost to the state will be much higher. First, treating illnesses that could have been prevented or identified at an earlier stage will entail significant cost. For example, the lifetime medical costs for one premature baby are conservatively estimated at $500,000. A recent study to quantify the lifetime cost of medical treatment for women younger than 65 with cardiovascular disease, diabetes or stress urinary incontinence, found the total lifetime cost of treatment is $233,000 more than the cost of treating someone without the condition.

Second, the impact on the dental safety net providers will be drastic. Over the last several years, the Federally Qualified Health Centers (FQHC), local public health departments, Schools of Dentistry, as well as the Michigan legislature have committed significant resources to increasing the availability of oral health providers willing to treat the Medicaid population. If we eliminate the reimbursement for serving the targeted population, many of these providers will experience practically a doubling of their uninsured populations. The mix of care provided by FQHCs to the uninsured and subsidized with federal grant dollars will likely shift more towards oral health services and will create a larger gap on the medical care side. Regardless of how uninsured care is financed, if at all, the funding will not double with the elimination of dental coverage. Instead, the providers will be forced to ration care. This will not only impact the health of the un-served population but will jeopardize the financial viability of the providers.

Reinstatement of oral health benefits even after a year of no funding will carry substantial redevelopment costs.

- Jobs will be eliminated.
- Facilities and equipment will be underutilized.
- People will unlearn the positive healthcare seeking habits developed with considerable safety net provider effort over the last several years.

Reinstatement of oral health benefits even after a year of no funding will carry substantial redevelopment costs.

> ***"American students miss millions of hours of school and adults miss millions of hours of work each year due to dental disease or visits. By improving our nation's oral health, we improve our nation's overall health."***
> ***-Surgeon General Richard Carmona***

The third major unintended consequence is the increase in costs associated with delayed treatment in the most expensive and usually inappropriate setting, the hospital emergency room. Hospitals that have evaluated the impact of oral health access problems have found substantial amounts of resources spent providing care to persons who present in their emergency rooms with untreated dental problems. In Muskegon, one hospital saw 2,400 dental related emergencies within 7 months this year alone. That accounts for 11.2 encounters a day even with two FQHCs serving the community. The two FQHCs employ a combined 5 FTE dentists and provided 24,591 oral health encounters in 2002. Inappropriate use of hospital emergency rooms will only worsen when adult oral health benefits are eliminated. Researchers found that after the state eliminated oral health benefits for beneficiaries in 1993, dental related claims in physicians' offices declined by 8%, and dental-related care in emergency departments increases 12% (American Journal of Public Health, August 2003). Many adults assumed they could not see their physicians nor their dentist when Medicaid dental services were cut. As a result, primary care access is reduced: The impact of eliminating the oral health benefit goes beyond "just dental."

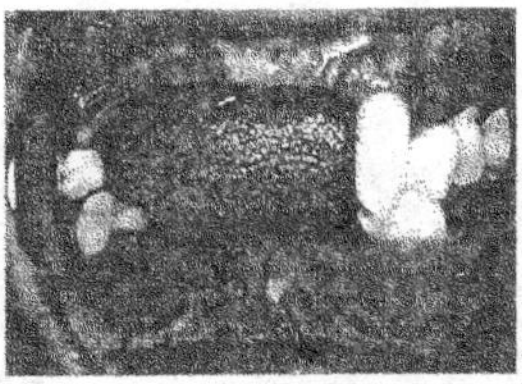

Finally, the impact on the patient's finances and family is too often devastating both due to time missed from work and inability to care for their children. Adults with poor oral health (i.e. unsightly smiles) face serious barriers to achieving full-time employment and have limited types of employment options. How many costumers want to order food from someone missing teeth (the only oral health treatment available to adults on Medicaid after October 1, 2003)? Oral diseases not only impact economic productivity, but can compromise our ability to work at home or at school, or on the job. Oral diseases affect our ability to eat, the foods we choose, and how we communicate. In straight economic terms, perhaps we should "put our money where are mouths are" [Quote from Dr. Elizabeth Duke, Administrator for Health Resources and Services Administration: NACHC Annual Convention, August 26, 2003].

We made a mistake. We have eliminated health for a vital part of the body. As a group, the administration, legislature, and advocates need to admit a mistake was made and decide how Michigan is going to rectify the situation. There are no easy answers but together we can make some critical and creative decisions.

The Michigan Primary Care Association and Michigan Association for Local Public Healthwelcome the opportunity to discuss the Reinstatement of Adult Oral Health Benefits for Medicaid Adults. Please feel free to contact any of those listed below.

Kim Sibilsky
Executive Director
MPCA
(517) 381-8000, ext. 211
ksibilsky@mpca.net

Carol Parker Lee
Chief of Policy and Planning
MPCA
(517) 381-8000, ext. 205
cplee@mpca.net

Mark Bertler
Executive Director
MALPH
(517) 485-0660
mbertler@malph.org

***Please note the attached bibliography referencing the vast amount of evidence based information available on the correlation between oral health and systemic health.**

Inequality in America: The Contribution of Health Centers in Reducing and Eliminating Disparities in Access to Care

Robert M. Politzer
Jean Yoon
Leiyu Shi
Ronda G. Hughes
Jerrilynn Regan
Marilyn H. Gaston

Reprinted from Medical Care Research and Review
Volume 58 No. 2, June 2001, pp. 234-248

Persistent and widening health care access and health status disparities (Center for Disease Control 1999) are particularly disturbing as evidence emerges that links access to a usual and regular source of primary care with improvements in health status, regardless of income (Shi and Starfield 2001). It has been argued that health care access can contribute only marginally to reducing or eliminating these disparities when facing formidable opposition from lack of education, poverty, and poor social environment (Williams 1999; Wilkinson 1997; Kennedy, Kawachi, and Prothrow-Stith 1996). Evidence indicates that access to primary care alone can mitigate health status disparities (Shi and Starfield 2001).

Internationally, there is concordance between the strength of a nation's primary care delivery system and its health status indicators (Starfield 1998). In studies within the United States, primary care was identified as the most significant medical care variable associated with better health status (Shi 1992; Farmer, Stokes, and Fisher 1991). One study demonstrated that primary care exerted a strong and significant influence on life expectancy and total mortality even after controlling for the adverse impact of income inequality (Shi et al. 1999). This study was replicated for U.S. metropolitan areas (Shi and Starfield 2001) and for several points in time (Shi and Starfield 2001) with similar results.

Other researchers have demonstrated the relationship between the performance of essential primary care functions and improved health status (Rosenblatt et al. 1998; Bunker, Frazier, and Mosteller 1994; Weiner and Starfield 1983). Studies have found that populations in geographic areas with higher family/general physician-to-population ratios had lower rates of avoidable hospitalization for Ambulatory Care Sensitive Conditions (ACSCs; Parchman and Culler 1994), and men appearing at emergency rooms with complications of hypertension were less likely to have a source of primary care than those without complications (Shea et al. 1992). Controlling for demographics and diagnoses, one study found that patients with a primary care physician as their personal physician had lower mortality than those with a specialist as their personal physician (Franks and Fiscella 1998). Finally, a recent study captured the domains of primary care (i.e., continuity, accessibility) and determined that quality primary care attenuates the adverse impact of income inequality on health (Shi and Starfield 2000).

The views expressed in this article are those of the authors and should not be inferred to the department or any of its components. We express our appreciation to Uma Gavarasana, M.D., a third year medical resident at Long Island Jewish Medical Center, New Hyde Park, NY, for her review and editing of this manuscript. This article, submitted to *Medical Care Research and Review* on July 19, 2000, was revised and accepted for publication on December 15, 2000.

NEW CONTRIBUTION

This article synthesizes results from the most recent literature in an attempt to establish the link between access to primary care and reductions in health status disparities. It presents the most up-to-date data on the performance and effectiveness of federally funded health centers in providing such access to primary care for vulnerable populations.

DATA COLLECTION METHOD

The BPHC has established a three-stage data collection activity to assess the effectiveness of health centers. At Stage 1, the Uniform Data System (UDS) collects a variety of financial, socioeconomic, demographic, and utilization information for every health center that receives federal support. Second, in 1995 a survey was launched of health center patients who had received care from a health center the previous year using an instrument comparable to the Center for Disease Control and Prevention's (CDC) National Health Interview Survey (NHIS). By using a similar tool and method, peer (i.e., adjusted for age, race, and socioeconomic status) comparison groups were created from the NHIS data. NHIS survey respondents were included only if they had at least one medical encounter with a health care professional. The health centers survey included patient demographics, insurance coverage, self-perceived health status, access to care, quality of care, patient satisfaction, activities of daily living, receipt of preventive services, and treatment of chronic conditions (for details on methodology, see Regan, Lefkowitz, and Gaston 1999). Finally, intensive studies were conducted of health center medical records and other databases (such as the Health Care Financing Administration's State Medicaid Research Files) to compare outcomes of health center patients with similar patients who obtained care from other sources.

RESULTS

HEALTH CENTER PATIENTS

An estimated 43 million people (1 in 6 Americans) live in federally designated underserved areas and lack access to a private primary care provider (Lefkowitz and Todd 1999). In 1998, 8.7 million people, one fifth of the 43

TABLE 1 Distribution of Health Center Patients by Race/Ethnicity, Income, and Insurance

	n	%
Race/ethnicity		
White	3,117,129	36
Hispanic	2,943,955	34
African American	2,251,259	26
Asian/other	346,347	4
Total	8,658,690	100
Income		
Below poverty	5,714,735	66
100% to 200% poverty	1,731,738	20
Below 200% poverty	1,212,217	14
Total	8,658,690	100
Type of insurance		
Uninsured	3,550,063	41
Medicaid	2,857,368	33
Medicare	606,108	7
Other/private	1,645,151	19
Total	8,658,690	100

Source: Adapted from the Bureau of Primary Health Care (1998).
Note: Income is defined according to the federal poverty guidelines. Below 200 percent poverty is $33,400 for a family of four in 1999. Unknown were distributed as known.

nation, African American health center patients have even higher rates; nearly half have hypertension, compared with 35 percent for low-income, adult African Americans (Mathematica Policy Research 1998b). Also, the prevalence of diabetes is higher among health center patients. This finding holds regardless of racial/ethnic group, income level, age, gender, or even among the obese. Even after controlling for risk factors such as obesity, race/ethnicity, and age, health center patients are significantly more likely to have the disease (Mathematica Policy Research 1998a).

About 7.1 percent of births to health center women are at or below 2,500 grams. This figure is comparable to the nation's, but health center women are more likely to be teenagers and from racial/ethnic minority groups with higher rates than the national average. African American women who use health centers give birth to low birth weight infants at a rate of 9.9 percent, in contrast to their national rate of 13.0 percent. Compared with national figures, health center rates represent a 50 percent reduction in this disparity.

(25 percent, 16 percent, and 12 percent, respectively) (BPHC, 1995). While 75 percent of the nation's uninsured reported having a usual source of care, 99 percent of health center uninsured reported having a usual source of care (Mathematica Policy Research 1999).

A study comparing pediatric visits to health centers with such visits to hospital-based primary care clinics and generalist office-based practices revealed that a greater percentage of health center visits were made by known patients returning for a new problem (odds ratios: 1.77 for health centers, 1.0 for offices, and 0.70 for clinics). Hospital-based clinics and generalist office-based practices, on the other hand, saw a greater percentage of known patients for old problems (Forrest and Whelan 2000; Whelan and Forrest 1999). Other researchers have demonstrated that the visit category "known patient for new problem" can be used as a proxy for continuity of care (Starfield 1998).

PREVENTION/SCREENING

Health center uninsured adults are more likely to receive counseling on lifestyle issues than uninsured adults who seek care elsewhere. Health center uninsured adults are more likely to be counseled about diet and eating habits (54 percent vs. 43 percent), physical activity (57 percent vs. 48.5 percent), smoking (75.4 percent vs. 63.9 percent), drinking (67.8 percent vs. 52.3 percent), drug use (55.2 percent vs. 38.7 percent), and sexually transmitted diseases (53.7 percent vs. 36.2 percent) than U.S. uninsured adults. However, in most cases the health center rate has not met the Healthy People 2000 goal, except for physical activity and tobacco use (Mathematica Policy Research 1999).

Pap smears, mammograms, and clinical breast examinations can detect disease in its early stages, significantly reducing morbidity and mortality. Even though the long-awaited decline in U.S. breast cancer mortality has arrived, the disparity between African American and white women persists (Chevarley and White 1997). One of the factors contributing to higher mortality for African American women is their higher likelihood of later stage diagnosis. Nationally, mammography rates for low-income women are below 50 percent across racial/ethnic groups and fall below the Healthy People 2000 goal of 60 percent (U.S. DHHS 1997). Yet for the 2.5 million health center women of childbearing age, their rates far exceed those of comparable women in the nation and meet or exceed the Healthy People 2000 goal (see Table 2).

For clinical breast examinations, health center women have rates around 80 percent, far exceeding the national rate for comparable women (62 percent). For up-to-date Pap smears, health center women not only exceed the national

TABLE 3 Health Center Screening by Race/Ethnicity (in percentages)

Race/Ethnicity	*Breast Exam*	*Mammogram*	*Pap Smear*	*Testicular Exam*	*Cholesterol Screening*
White	82	57	82	47	44
Non-white	79	64	84	48	46

Source: Adapted from Frick and Regan (2000).

TABLE 4 Up-to-Date Cancer Screening among Adult Health Center Women by Insurance Status (in percentages)

	Health Center[a]			*United States*[b]		
Insurance	*Pap Smear*	*Mammography*	*Breast Exam*	*Pap Smear*	*Mammography*	*Breast Exam*
Medicaid	93.4	65.6	88.0	41	38	52
Uninsured	88.2	55.9	79.0	32	19	38
Private/other insurance	91.6	56.2	83.1	58	55	62

Source: Adapted from Regan, Lefkowitz, and Gaston (1999) and Makuc, Freid, and Parsons (1994).
a. Pap smear within 1 to 3 years. Mammography and breast exams in the past 2 years.
b. Within the past year.

QUALITY OF CARE

Additional evidence of health center ability to provide access to appropriate care can be gleaned from its chronic disease management. Health center practices meet or significantly exceed literature-based standards for treatment of the most common conditions of hypertension, acute otitis media, diabetes, and asthma on over 80 percent of the care elements (Ulmer et al. 2000). Hypertensive health center African American and Hispanic patients report at a rate of 90 percent that their blood pressure is under control, more than three times that of a comparable group of hypertensives in the nation and nearly double the Healthy People 2000 goal of 50 percent (Mathematica Policy Research 1998b). Health center diabetics report that their glycohemoglobin rates are tested on schedule 43 percent of the time. Although this rate falls below the Healthy People 2000 goal of 60 percent, it is more than twice the rate reported in the literature (Mathematica Policy Research 1998a).

(Fiscella et al. 2000). Health centers will use the categories and subcategories currently advanced by the Bureau of the Census for its decenniel census.

Reducing the stubborn health care access and health status disparities of poor people from racial/ethnic minority groups and who are uninsured is a challenge to safety net providers (Rosenbaum et al. 2000; Institute of Medicine 2000). The results presented indicate the contribution of health centers in reducing these disparities, particularly the low birth weight disparity for African American infants and the racial/ethnic, income, and insurance status disparities for important preventive screening procedures. Health centers assist patients in obtaining and complying with care by providing interpreter services, cultural competence training, and targeted outreach programs, striving to serve as their patients' usual and regular source of primary care (Zuvekas, McNamara, and Bernstein 1999). The recorded improvements in health care access are likely to have an impact on health status.

Health centers serve 8.7 million of the approximately 43 million people without access to a private primary care provider, up from about 8.3 million in 1997. This pace is insufficient to meet the needs in a timely manner of the remaining 34 million living in underserved communities without access. As such, the nation needs a multipronged approach to achieve 100 percent access to primary care and narrow and eliminate the gap in health status.

First, it seems reasonable to continue to strengthen the existing health centers' safety net to assure that health care access and ultimately health status disparities among their patients are continually reduced and eventually eliminated. It also seems reasonable to expand existing networks to reach additional people currently without access. Finally, it remains a challenge to leverage scarce resources within communities of the remaining 34 million underserved to identify needs and develop systems that address those needs. Regardless of strategy or plan, the safety net of providers of care for vulnerable people needs to become their usual and regular source of care if the nation intends to reduce and eliminate health care access and health status disparities.

REFERENCES

Bunker, J., H. Frazier, and F. Mosteller. 1994. Improving health: Measuring the effects of medical care. *Milbank Quarterly* 72:225-28.

Bureau of Primary Health Care. 1995. *Health center user visit survey.* Bethesda, MD: Author.

———. 1998. *Uniform data system national summary data 1998.* June. Bethesda, MD: Author.

———. 1999. *FY 2001 budget presentation: Office of data, evaluation, analysis and research.* December. Bethesda, MD: Author.

Makuc, D. M., V. M. Freid, and P. E. Parsons. 1994. *Health insurance and cancer screening among women*. Advance data from vital and health statistics no. 254. Hyattsville, MD: National Center for Health Statistics.

Mathematica Policy Research. 1998a. *Profile of diabetics from health center user/visit survey: Final report*. November. Bethesda, MD: Bureau of Primary Health Care.

———. 1998b. *Profile of hypertensives from health center user/visit survey: Final report*. December. Bethesda, MD: Bureau of Primary Health Care.

———.1999. *Profile of uninsured from health center user/visit survey: Final report*. February. Bethesda, MD: Bureau of Primary Health Care.

National Center for Health Statistics. 1991. *Public use data file documentation: Linked birth/infant death data set: 1991 birth cohort*. Hyattsville, MD: Author.

Parchman, M. L., and S. Culler. 1994. Primary care physicians and avoidable hospitalizations. *Journal of Family Practice* 39 (2): 123-28.

Regan, J., B. Lefkowitz, and M. Gaston. 1999. Cancer screening among community health center women: Eliminating the gaps. *Journal of Ambulatory Care Management* 22 (4): 45-52.

Rosenbaum, S., P. Shu, A. Markus, and J. Darnell. 2000. *Health centers role as safety net providers for Medicaid patients and the uninsured*. Kaiser Commission on Medicaid and the Uninsured, February.

Rosenblatt, R., L. Hart, L. Baldwin, L. Chan, and R. Schneeweiss. 1998. The generalist role of specialty physicians: Is there a hidden system of primary care? *Journal of American Medical Association* 279:1364-70.

Shea, S., D. Misra, M. H. Ehrlich, L. Field, and C. K. Francis. 1992. Predisposing factors for severe, uncontrolled hypertension in an inner-city minority population. *New England Journal of Medicine* 327:776-81.

Shi, L. 1992. The relation between primary care and life chances. *Journal of Health Care for the Poor and Underserved* 2:321-35.

Shi, L., and B. Starfield. 2000. Primary care, income inquality and racial mortality in metropolitan areas. *American Journal of Public Health* (forthcoming).

———. 2000. Primary care, income inequality, and self-rated health in the U.S.: Mixed level analysis. *International Journal of Health Services* 30:541-45.

Shi, L., B. Starfield, B. Kennely, and I. Kavachi. 1999. Income inequality, primary care and health indicators. *Journal of Family Practice* 48:275-84.

Starfield, B. 1998. *Primary care, balancing health needs, services, and technology*. New York: Oxford University Press.

Ulmer, C., D. Lewis-Idema, A. Von Worley, J. Rodgers, L. B. Berger, E. J. Darling, and B. Lefkowitz. 2000. Assessing primary care content: Four conditions common in community health center practice. *Journal of Ambulatory Care Management* 23 (1): 23-38.

U.S. Census Bureau. 1999. *Health insurance coverage 1998*. U.S. Department of Commerce, P60-208, October.

LexisNexis

Lab Business Week

February 27, 2005

SECTION: EXPANDED REPORTING; Pg. 199

LENGTH: 917 words

HEADLINE: STATE **MEDICAID;**
Medicaid programs enticing to states with budget problems

BODY:

Disabled and unable to work, David Kuehl put off dental care for 6 years. After becoming eligible for **Medicaid,** he had several damaged teeth removed to ward off the infections he's prone to as a hemophiliac.

Medicaid coverage for adult dental services, which survived budget cutting 2 years ago, is back in the mix as Governor Bob Taft and lawmakers say they need to look for savings everywhere in a spending plan already facing a $5 billion deficit.

Across the country, programs considered optional under **Medicaid** rules are enticing as states wrestle with stagnant revenue and soaring healthcare costs. The National Governors Association calls **Medicaid** reform its top priority this year.

"What's a word bigger than catastrophe?" said Barb Edwards, deputy director of Ohio's **Medicaid** program.

Kuehl, of Buckland in western Ohio, said he couldn't have afforded the $20,000-plus in treatment, which included a hospital stay, without **Medicaid,** which covered everything. And as a hemophiliac, he is subject to uncontrolled bleeding from even minor injuries or infections.

"Not only is it a financial burden, but it would also put my life at risk," the 48-year-old former maintenance worker said.

In the past 3 years, several states reduced adult dental coverage under **Medicaid** for budget reasons, including Michigan, Minnesota and Utah. In California, Connecticut, New Jersey and other states, intense lobbying by dentists blocked similar moves.

The number of states with comprehensive dental benefits for adults under **Medicaid** dropped to seven in 2004, down from 14 in 2000, according to an analysis by the American Dental Association.

In 2003, Minnesota added a $500 cap to dental services that don't include major procedures like extractions, saving about $1 million a year, said Brian Osberg, the state's assistant commissioner of healthcare.

As a result, some patients are choosing to have all their teeth pulled and replaced by dentures, which **Medicaid** still covers, rather than the less invasive procedures which they can't afford, said Richard Diercks, executive director of the Minnesota Dental Association.

The change was necessary because of state budget problems, and the cap was better than no dental coverage at all, said Republican state Representative Tim Wilkin.

Advocates for the poor say reducing the benefits would hurt the needy and cost states more in the long run because patients dropped may seek more costly emergency treatment.

Dentists and others also argue that poor dental health can lead to additional health problems, including diabetes, strokes and premature births in women.

"It is really foolish to not provide those preventative and acute care programs for adults, because some of the most expensive conditions are exacerbated by oral health problems," said Shelly Gehshan, a program director with the National Conference of State Legislatures.

At stake in Ohio is about $28 million from the state and $42 million in matching federal funds. The money covers everything from routine office visits, at costs starting at an average of $45, to major surgery.

About 247,000 Ohio adults on **Medicaid,** or about 31%, used a dental service at least once during 2003.

The potential loss comes at a time when access to dental care is considered by the Ohio Health Department as one of the state's top unmet medical needs.

Taft will introduce a budget in February that tries to keep the growth in **Medicaid,** the state-federal program for poor children and families, to about 4% a year. It's no small task for a $10.5 billion program that ran double-digit increases from 2001 through 2004.

The Republican governor warned last fall that increases in **Medicaid,** which could account for up to 40% of state spending over the next 2 years, must be slowed.

Reductions in dental funding are being watched closely by **community health centers,** which often serve children and adults on **Medicaid.**

"Almost every state we're aware of that was providing dental for adults as an optional service has dropped it or is thinking about it," said Roger Schwartz, state affairs director for the National Association of **Community Health Centers.**

In North Carolina, lawmakers tried unsuccessfully in 2002 to reduce funding to the state's dental program. Dentists fear the state may try again for budget reasons.

"Adults need to be able to get a job, they need to be able to be healthy," said Cynthia Bolton, MD, a dentist in Reidsville, North Carolina. "You certainly can't interview well for a job if you don't have your teeth."

Lawmakers have tough funding decisions to make, and optional services are a possibility, said Ohio Representative Shawn Webster, a Millville Republican who was chairman of a state committee studying ways to reduce **Medicaid** costs.

"You look at what you have to spend your money on first, and then you fund that, and if you have money left over, then you look at optional services," he said.

At the East Central Health Clinic in a poor Columbus neighborhood, two dentists and two dental assistants serve a steady mix of the homeless, the uninsured and those on **Medicaid.**

"I wish I could find whoever called dental an optional service," said clinic director David Heisel.

"I wish they could be in the same circumstances, have no money, have a swollen painful face, and no place to go," Heisel said. "Then I don't think they'd consider it optional."

LOAD-DATE: February 18, 2005

2004 National Healthcare Disparities Report

U.S. Department of Health and Human Services

Agency for Healthcare Research and Quality
540 Gaither Road
Rockville, MD 20850

AHRQ Publication No. 05-0014
December 2004

Second Printing, March 2005

Acknowledgments

The National Healthcare Disparities Report (NHDR) is the product of collaboration among agencies across the Department of Health and Human Services (HHS). Many individuals guided and contributed to this report. Without their wisdom and magnanimous support, this report would not have been possible.

Specifically, we thank:

Primary AHRQ Staff: Carolyn Clancy, Daniel Stryer, Katherine Crosson, Ernest Moy, Elizabeth Dayton, Karen Ho, and Donna Rae Castillo.

HHS Advisors: Hakan Aykan (ASPE), Agnes Davidson (OSOPHS), Ruth Katz (ASPE), and Marty McGeein (ASPE).

HHS Interagency Work Group for the NHDR: Irma Arispe (CDC-NCHS), Felicia Collins (HRSA), Martin Dannenfelser (ACF), Emily DeVoto (NIH), Tuei Doong (OSOPHS), Latecia Engram (HRSA), Brenda Evelyn (FDA), Anita Everett (SAMHSA), Saadia Greenberg (AoA), Tom Hertz (ASPE), Deloris Hunter (NIH), Richard Klein (CDC-NCHS), Te ry Lied (CMS), Leopold Luberecki (ASL), Diane Makuc (CDC-NCHS), Saralyn Mark (OSOPHS), Susan Queen (HRSA), Beatrice Rouse (SAMHSA), Phillip Smith (IHS), Benedict Truman (CDC), Nadarajen Vydelingum (NIH), Valerie Welsh (OSOPHS), and Dinah Wiley (OCR).

AHRQ NHDR Data Group: E mest Moy, chair, Roxanne Andrews, Sepheen Byron, Kaytura Felix-Aaron, Edward Kelley, Gary Olin, Sari Siegel, and Marc Zodet.

AHRQ Center for Quality Improvement and Patient Safety NHQR/NHDR Team: Edward Kelley, director, James Burgdorf, Elizabeth Dayton, Tina Ding, Diana Dodd, Darryl Gray, Karen Ho, Kelly McDermott, Dwight McNeill, Ernest Moy, Anna Poker, Judy Sangl, David Stevens, and Chunliu Zhan.

HHS Data Experts: Barbara Bartman (HRSA), Steven Cohen (AHRQ), Karen Edrington (CMS), Paul Eggers (NIH), Trena Ezzati-Rice (AHRQ), John Fleishman (AHRQ), Diane Frankenfield (CMS), Reem Ghandour (HRSA), Joe Gfroerer (SAMHSA), Julia Holmes (CDC-NCHS), Edwin Huff (CMS), Kenneth Keppel (CDC-NCHS), Doris Lefkowitz (AHRQ), Suzanne Proctor (CDC-NCHS), Lynn Ries (NIH), and Colleen Ryan Smith (IHS), and Todd Wilson (CDC).

Other AHRQ Contributors: Fran Chevarley, Rosaly Correa, Carole, Denise Dougherty, Sharon Larson, Pamela Owens, Larry Patton, Denise Remus, Mary Rolston, Randie Siegel, and Phyllis Zucker. AHRQ would also like to acknowledge the contributions of the late Ellen Howe in support of NHDR activities.

Contents

Key Themes and Highlights From the National Healthcare Disparities Report

The United States health care delivery system is among the world's finest with outstanding providers, facilities, and technology. Many Americans enjoy easy access to care. However, not all Americans have full access to high quality health care.

Released in 2003, the first National Healthcare Disparities Report (NHDR) is a comprehensive national overview of disparities in health care among racial, ethnic, and socioeconomic groups in the general U.S. population and among priority populations. This second NHDR is built upon the 2003 report and continues to include a comprehensive national overview of disparities in health care in America. In addition, in the 2004 report, a second critical goal of the report is developed: tracking the Nation's progress towards the elimination of health care disparities.

In the 2004 report, three key themes are highlighted for policymakers, clinicians, health system administrators, and community leaders who seek to use this information to improve health care services for all Americans:

- Disparities are pervasive.
- Improvement is possible.
- Gaps in information exist, especially for specific conditions and populations.

Disparities Are Pervasive

Consistent with extensive research and findings in the 2003 report, the 2004 report finds that disparities related to race, ethnicity, and socioeconomic status[i] pervade the American health care system. While varying in magnitude by condition and population, disparities are observed in almost all aspects of health care, including:

- Across all dimensions of quality of health care including effectiveness, patient safety, timeliness, and patient centeredness.
- Across all dimensions of access to care including getting into the health care system, getting care within the health care system, patient perceptions of care, and health care utilization.
- Across many levels and types of care including preventive care, acute care, and chronic care.
- Across many clinical conditions including cancer, diabetes, end stage renal disease, heart disease, and respiratory diseases.
- Across many care settings including primary care, dental care, mental health care, substance abuse treatment, emergency rooms, hospitals, and nursing homes.
- Within many subpopulations including women, children, elderly, persons with disabilities, residents of rural areas, and individuals with special health care needs.

[i]Consistent with Healthy People 2010, the NHDR defines disparities as any differences among populations. In addition, all disparities discussed in the NHDR meet criteria based on statistical significance and size of difference described in Chapter 1. Income and education are the primary measures of socioeconomic status used in the report.

To begin to quantify disparities systematically, a subset of measures for which comparable data are available for 2000 and 2001 are highlighted in the 2004 report. This subset consists of 38 measures of effectiveness of health care and 31 measures of access to health care. Data sources are the Surveillance, Epidemiology, and End Results (SEER) program, U.S. Renal Data System (USRDS), Medical Expenditure Panel Survey (MEPS), the Centers for Disease Control and Prevention (CDC) AIDS Surveillance System, National Vital Statistics System-Natality (NVSS-N), National Immunization Survey (NIS), National Health Interview Survey (NHIS), and National Hospital Discharge Survey (NHDS). For each measure, racial, ethnic, and socioeconomic groups are compared with an appropriate comparison group; each group could receive care that is poorer than, about the same as, or better than the comparison group.[ii] For each group, the percentage of measures for which the group received poorer care was then calculated.

Figure H.1. Percent of measures for which members of selected racial groups experience poorer quality of care (left) or have worse access to care (right) compared with whites in 2000 and 2001

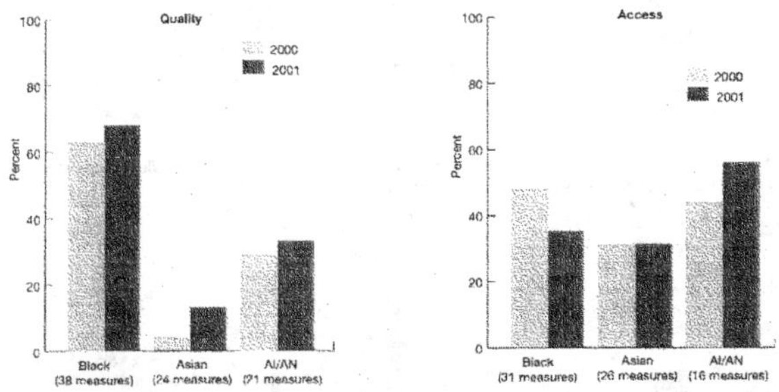

Source: SEER, USRDS, MEPS, CDC AIDS Surveillance System, NVSS-N, NIS, NHIS, NHDS, 2000-2001.

Note: Poorer quality of care and worse access to care indicate that for a particular measure, the group does not receive as high quality care or have as much access to care as whites and that the relative difference is at least 10% and statistically significant with $p<0.05$. Number of measures available for each group is indicated in parentheses.

Key: AI/AN=American Indian and Alaska Native

Of measures tracked in 2000 and 2001, in both years:

- Blacks received poorer quality of care than whites for about two-thirds of quality measures and had worse access to care than whites for about 40% of access measures (Figure H.1).
- Asians[iii] received poorer quality of care than whites for about 10% of quality measures and had worse access to care than whites for about a third of access measures.
- American Indians and Alaska Natives (AI/ANs) received poorer quality of care than whites for about a third of quality measures and had worse access to care than whites for about half of access measures.

[ii] Data on all measures were not available for all groups; see Tables 1.2 and 1.3 for lists of measures available for each group. Only relative differences of at least 10% and statistically significant with $p< 0.05$ are discussed in this report.

[iii] Including "Asians or Pacific Islanders (APIs)" when information is not collected separately for each group.

Figure H.2. Percent of measures for which Hispanics experience poorer quality of care (left) or have worse access to care (right) compared with non-Hispanic whites in 2000 and 2001

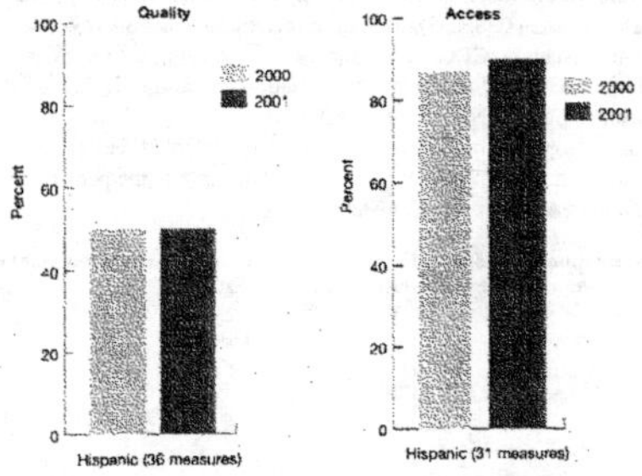

Source: SEER, USRDS, MEPS, CDC AIDS Surveillance System, NVSS-N, NIS, NHIS, NHDS, 2000-2001.

Note: Poorer quality of care and worse access to care indicate that for a particular measure, the group does not receive as high quality care or have as much access to care as non-Hispanic whites and that the relative difference is at least 10% and statistically significant with $p<0.05$. Number of measures available for each group is indicated in parentheses.

Figure H.3. Percent of measures for which the poor experience poorer quality of care (left) or have worse access to care (right) compared with high income individuals in 2000 and 2001

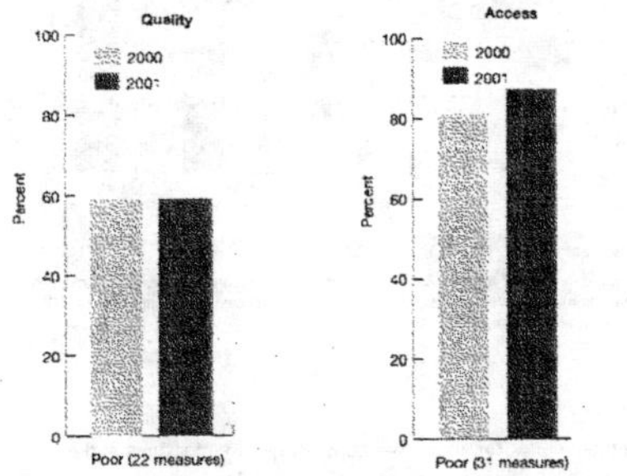

Source: SEER, USRDS, MEPS, CDC AIDS Surveillance System, NVSS-N, NIS, NHIS, NHDS, 2000-2001.

Note: Poorer quality of care and worse access to care indicate that for a particular measure, the group does not receive as high quality care or have as much access to care as high income individuals and that the relative difference is at least 10% and statistically significant with $p<0.05$. Number of measures available for each group is indicated in parentheses.

Of measures tracked in 2000 and 2001, in both years:

- Hispanics received lower quality of care than non-Hispanic whites for half of quality measures and had worse access to care than non-Hispanic whites for about 90% of access measures (Figure H.2).
- Poor people[iv] received lower quality of care for about 60% of quality measures and had worse access to care for about 80% of access measures than those with high income (Figure H.3).

[iv] "Poor" is defined as having family incomes less than 100% of the Federal poverty level and "high income" is defined as having family incomes 400% or more of the Federal poverty level.

Improvement Is Possible

The Department of Health and Human Services (HHS) leads many initiatives aimed at reducing health care disparities and improving health care quality. While cause and effect relationships would be difficult to demonstrate, these activities are often associated with improvements in care. In the 2003 report, several examples of the absence or reversal of disparity that coincided with HHS programs were identified, including:

- Absence of racial or ethnic disparity in management of anemia among end stage renal disease patients in 2001, coinciding with the Centers for Medicare & Medicaid Services End Stage Renal Disease Clinical Performance Measures Project.
- Higher rates of Pap testing among black compared with white women in 2000, coinciding with the CDC National Breast and Cervical Cancer Early Detection Program.
- Higher rates of blood pressure monitoring among blacks compared with whites in 1998, coinciding with the National Heart, Lung, and Blood Institute National High Blood Pressure Education Program.

In the 2004 report, new examples of decreasing disparities in health care are added, including:

- Elimination of racial, ethnic, and socioeconomic disparities in quality of and access to health care observed among people who receive care in community health centers.
- Elimination of differences in rates of late stage breast cancer between black and white women from 1992 to 2001 due to falling rates among black women coupled with rising rates among white women. This result may be related to the CDC National Breast and Cervical Cancer Early Detection Program and improving rates of mammography among black women.
- Lower rates of measles-mumps-rubella vaccination for black children age 19-35 months compared with white children and lower rates of *Haemophilus influenzae* vaccination for Hispanic children compared with non-Hispanic white children in 2000 but no significant differences in 2002. These results may in part be related to the CDC National Immunization Program.
- Lower rates of influenza vaccination for elderly Asian and Pacific Islander Medicare beneficiaries than white beneficiaries in 1998 but no significant difference in 2000.
- Less likelihood that blacks and Asians would report a source of ongoing care compared with whites in 1999 but no significant differences in 2001.

While these examples demonstrate that improvement is possible, reducing disparities is a gradual process. In the 2004 report, the accumulation of more than a single year of data for many measures allows the examination of changes over time. While changes over 2 years of data are difficult to interpret, these changes are presented in this report to illustrate the tracking function of the NHDR. It is hoped that future reports with more years of data will be able to document sustained reductions in health care disparities.

In general, from one year to the next, improvements in measures of quality of or access to health care are small, and disparities are particularly slow to change. For all racial, ethnic, and socioeconomic groups, specific disparities observed in 2000 were almost always observed in 2001 as well (Figures H.1-H.3). Even when improvement in quality or access is observed, disparities often persist because all groups typically change proportionately. To reduce disparities, groups with poorer quality of care or access to care need to experience more rapid improvement in care than other groups and this is rarely observed.

Longer term trends are better able to capture improvements in health care over time but generally support the thesis that disparities changegradually. For example, the three SEER measures used in the report are trended over a decade. For two of these, significant changes over the decade are demonstrated; rates of late stage colorectal and cervical cancer fell while rates of late stage breast cancer remained constant. However, most of the racial and ethnic differences in late stage cancer observed in 1992 are still present in 2001.

Gaps in Information Exist, Especially for Specific Conditions and Populations

In the 2003 report, providing a comprehensive national overview of disparities in health care was limited by a number of gaps in information, including:

- Few measures for some conditions such as quality of HIV care and mental health care.
- Few measures that were unique but important to specific populations.
- Limited data to address particular population groups such as children, the elderly, persons with disabilities, residents of rural areas, and individuals with special health care needs or at the end of life.
- Limited data to address Hispanic and Asian subpopulations and barriers related to language and literacy.
- Limited data to understand why disparities exist and how they can be eliminated.

In the 2004 report, efforts to address some of these information gaps have begun, including:

- More measures of unique and high importance to children and to the elderly.
- Information about hospital care received by American Indians and Alaska Natives from Indian Health Service facilities.
- Information about care delivered in community health centers from the Health Resources and Services Administration Community Health Center User Survey.
- Information about children with special health care needs from the National Survey of Children with Special Health Care Needs.
- Expanded analyses of residents along the urban-rural continuum using the new Federal classification system.
- Expanded stratified and multivariate analyses that begin to disaggregate disparities related to race and ethnicity from disparities related to socioeconomic status.

However, many gaps in information remain. For example, of the subset of measures tracked between 2000 and 2001, statistically reliable estimates were not possible for:

- The vast majority of measures among Native Hawaiians and Other Pacific Islanders.
- About half of measures among American Indians and Alaska Natives.
- About a third of quality of care measures among Asians.

Future NHDRs will benefit from ever improving data for examining and tracking disparities. For example, MEPS data for the 2005 report will include large oversamples of Asians and people with incomes less than 200% of the Federal poverty level and will add new survey questions about language and cultural competency. NHIS data will also begin to include oversamples of Asians. The increasing number of health plans that are beginning to collect data on race and ethnicity will improve understanding of disparities in health care. The revolution in health information technologies will allow data needed to assess disparities to be collected and processed more quickly, efficiently, securely, and economically.

As knowledge of disparities in health care and commitment to reducing disparities continue to grow, the ability to monitor and track improvements in disparities will become critical. In the 2004 report, work begun in 2003 to lay the information infrastructure needed to track the Nation's progress towards the elimination of disparities in health care is continued and expanded. Working together, using the NHDR as a guide, America's patients, providers, purchasers, and policymakers can make full access to high quality health care a reality for all.

Figure 27

Medicaid Acute Care Services

Mandatory Services

- Physician, nurse practitioner and nurse midwife services
- Laboratory and x-ray services
- Inpatient and outpatient hospital services
- Screening and treatment services for children (EPSDT)
- Family planning services
- Federally-qualified health center (FQHC) and rural health clinic (RHC) services

Optional Services

- Prescribed drugs
- Medical care or remedial care furnished by licensed practitioners under state law
- Diagnostic, screening, preventive, and rehabilitative services
- Clinic services
- Dental services, dentures
- Physical therapy and related services
- Prosthetic devices
- Eyeglasses
- TB-related services
- Primary care case management services
- Other specified medical and remedial care

Source: Kaiser Commission on Medicaid and the Uninsured, "The Medicaid Resource Book", July 2002

DEPARTMENT OF HEALTH & HUMAN SERVICES

Health Resources and Services Administration

Rockville MD 20857

AUG 17 2005

The Honorable John Dingell
House of Representatives
Washington, D.C. 20515

Dear Mr. Dingell:

Thank you for your inquiries for the record transmitted to me by Mr. Whitfield, Chairman, Subcommittee on Oversight and Investigations, Committee on Energy and Commerce.

I enjoyed the opportunity to testify at the Subcommittee on Oversight and Investigations Hearing on May 25, 2005, entitled: "A Review of Community Health Centers: Issues and Opportunities."

Enclosed, please find the text of the questions you posed and my responses. I hope this information is helpful. Please let me know if I can be of further assistance.

Sincerely,

Elizabeth M. Duke
Administrator

Enclosure

The Committee on Energy and Commerce
Subcommittee on Oversight and Investigations
"A Review of Community Health Centers: Issues and Opportunities"
May 25, 2005 – Questions for the Record

Questions from the Honorable John D. Dingell

1. In FY 2005, Congress provided almost $1.75 billion for community health centers. Several programs of the Bureau of Primary Health Care will be, or have been, delayed in the current fiscal year, so the Bureau may actually be funding those programs with FY 2006 money. Would you explain how the FY 2005 funding for community health centers has been or is being allocated? Will the Bureau continue to forward fund 330 grant programs?

   Answer: No funding for HRSA programs has been delayed or moved into subsequent fiscal years. In fact, HRSA has awarded all of the program dollars that have been appropriated, to date. However, when current fiscal year funds were exhausted, HRSA pre-approved some FY 2005 applications for future funding (see answer to question #3) based on the availability of FY 2006 funds.

   The increased appropriation provided for the Health Centers program in FY 2005 has enabled HRSA to move closer to the target of the President's Initiative of creating 1,200 new or expanded health center sites by FY 2006. Competitive review cycles were carried out to add 93 New Access Points (NAP) and 64 expanded capacity sites. In addition, 22 grantees were awarded grants for service expansion. Congress also provided funds to award approximately $31 million to existing grantees for a base adjustment.

   In order to achieve a wide distribution of NAP awards in FY 2005, HRSA considered the following factors:

   - Rural/Urban Distribution Of Awards: Aggregate awards in FY 2005 to serve rural and urban areas were made to ensure that no more than 60 percent and no fewer than 40 percent of the people served come from either rural or urban areas.
   - Proportionate Distribution: Aggregate awards in FY 2005 to support the various types of health centers were made to ensure continued proportionate distribution of funds across the Consolidated Health Center Program.
   - Geographic Consideration: The goal of HRSA is to expand the current safety net on a national basis by creating new access points in areas not currently served by a funded health center. Therefore, HRSA considered geographic distribution when deciding which applications to fund.

2. How will the delay of program announcements affect the President's commitment to open or expand 1,200 center sites by 2006?

Answer: There will be no effect on the ability to reach the goals of the President's Health Center Initiative by the end of 2006 caused by any delay in issuing application guidances. Regardless of the timing for publication of these guidances, HRSA has successfully awarded funding to support new and expanded sites since 2002.

3. Is it accurate that the 2004 New Access Point grants were delayed and then made with 2005 money?

   Answer: Yes, the FY 2004 appropriation funded 48 FY 2003 applications and 15 FY 2004 applications for a total of 63 NAPs funded with FY 2004 funding. Of the FY 2004 applications, 76 New Access Point applications were delayed and funded early in FY 2005 after the Consolidated Health Center program received a final appropriation that included funds for additional new access points.

   In fact, both the House and Senate Appropriations Committee Report language has supported the long-standing HRSA policy of approving specific qualified applications for future funding. This process has enabled high-quality applicants to take steps to develop and implement care delivery systems in their communities instead of wasting scarce resources to reapply for funding.

4. If, as numerous studies have found, community health centers provide better care for less money and actually cut Medicaid spending, why are we not funding even more centers? Would that not be a way to reduce Medicaid spending without cutting off beneficiaries?

   Answer: Studies show that Medicaid patients who received primary health care at health centers are less likely to be hospitalized for potentially avoidable conditions than beneficiaries who receive care elsewhere. In addition, research shows that Medicaid patients served by health centers are less likely to use the emergency room than Medicaid patients who are not served by health centers.

   The President has recognized the importance of health centers and in FY 2002 launched his Health Centers Initiative to create 1,200 new or expanded health center sites to serve an additional 6.1 million people by 2006. To achieve this goal, the President's Budget has requested yearly increases in funding for health centers from FY 2002 – FY 2006. Appropriations have increased over the same period, although in FY 2004 and FY 2005 the appropriated amounts were less than the President's requests. Below is a table listing the President's request and the appropriation.

Health Center Funding (in billions of dollars)					
	FY 2002	FY 2003	FY 2004	FY 2005	FY 2006
President's Budget*	1.289	1.434	1.582	1.791	1.967^
Appropriation*	1.328	1.465	1.573	1.690	1.764

*Does not include Federal Tort Claims Act funding

^The President's FY 2006 request includes an additional $26 million to fund new health centers in high-poverty counties.

DEPARTMENT OF HEALTH & HUMAN SERVICES

Health Resources and Services Administration

Rockville MD 20857

AUG 17 2005

The Honorable Tammy Baldwin
House of Representatives
Washington, D.C. 20515

Dear Ms. Baldwin:

Thank you for your inquiries for the record transmitted to me by Mr. Whitfield, Chairman, Subcommittee on Oversight and Investigations, Committee on Energy and Commerce.

I enjoyed the opportunity to testify at the Subcommittee on Oversight and Investigations Hearing on May 25, 2005, entitled: "A Review of Community Health Centers: Issues and Opportunities."

Enclosed, please find the text of the questions you posed and my responses. I hope this information is helpful. Please let me know if I can be of further assistance.

Sincerely,

Elizabeth M. Duke
Administrator

Enclosure

The Committee on Energy and Commerce
Subcommittee on Oversight and Investigations
"A Review of Community Health Centers: Issues and Opportunities"
May 25, 2005 – Questions for the Record

Questions from the Honorable Tammy Baldwin

1. My understanding is when Federally Qualified Health Centers (FQHCs) receive a Section 330 grant, HRSA requires some of the funds be used to ensure the FQHC has the capability of providing dental services. However, as you know, some States have opted to not include dental services under their Medicaid program. Without Medicaid reimbursement of dental services, some FQHCs cannot afford to provide dental services. Therefore, the dental suites that were built are not used.

   Do you believe that this requirement should be reevaluated since States are struggling to maintain their current Medicaid programs, and Federal cuts to Medicaid have been proposed?

   Answer: Currently, all New Access Point applications must demonstrate that all persons will have ready access to the full range of required primary, preventive, enabling and supplemental health services, including oral health care, mental health care and substance abuse services, either directly on-site or through established arrangements without regard to ability to pay. All States, currently, are required to provide dental services for children under 18 as part of the Medicaid EPSDT program. It has been documented in the Surgeon General's Report on Oral Health that there are significant oral health status disparities in low-income populations eligible for Medicaid. Health Centers should continue to demonstrate that access to care is available, either by providing services or by contracting with other referral providers.

   Very few recently funded dental programs have dental suites that are not used. Most health centers that have dental programs are working at or near capacity. The need for care is still tremendous for working poor and families at or below poverty. Eliminating the requirement to provide oral health care could potentially result in a significant increase in utilization of hospital emergency rooms, thus driving up cost to States and communities, while patients receive ineffective or inappropriate care.

2. Do community health centers provide HIV/AIDS testing and HIV/AIDS care and treatment? It seems to me that these centers, located in both urban and rural areas, are perfect places to conduct HIV testing. Are community health centers routinely offering HIV tests to people coming through their doors? And, if a person does test positive, what do they do next for them so that they can receive proper care and treatment?

   As you know, HIV/AIDS care and treatment is highly specialized and requires highly trained medical providers and continued patient testing and monitoring. In addition, many HIV/AIDS patients require a high degree of attention, and we are blessed with the Ryan White CARE Act, which provides many of these valuable life saving services that can not be easily replaced. Do you see a difference between the health care that community health centers offer and those offered under the Ryan White CARE Act?

Answer: Currently (2004), nearly 93 percent of the health centers report that they provide HIV testing and counseling on site. Health centers actually conducted nearly 425,000 HIV tests in 2004 on more than 375,000 patients. About 73,000 patients, generating over 390,000 encounters, received a primary diagnosis of symptomatic or asymptomatic HIV infection.

If a person tests positive for HIV, health centers follow appropriate clinical protocols based on the patient's diagnosis, viral load, and HIV status. The level of care ranges from appropriate referral to an HIV specialist in a community and co-management between the specialist and the health center. Many health centers have the capacity and staff to provide comprehensive HIV care within the health center.

The HIV/AIDS epidemic has profoundly affected the populations traditionally served by HRSA funded programs. In recent years, HIV/AIDS medical care has shifted increasingly towards primary care and outpatient management. Health centers are responding by addressing HIV/AIDS as a chronic disease in order to improve quality of services and eliminate the health disparities affecting people living with HIV/AIDS.

The HIV/AIDS Bureau, which manages the funding program for the Ryan White CARE Act, and the Bureau of Primary Health Care Health Center Program are both part of HRSA. In 2003, there were 171 health centers that were dually funded by these HRSA programs. There is no significant difference in HIV care in those health centers that also are funded by Ryan White programs. Most health centers that do not receive Ryan White funding provide access to testing, counseling, and some form of HIV care support either within the health center itself or by referral.

DEPARTMENT OF HEALTH & HUMAN SERVICES

Centers for Medicare & Medicaid Services

200 Independence Avenue SW
Washington, DC 20201

SEP 16

The Honorable Ed Whitfield, Chairman
Energy and Commerce Subcommittee on Oversight and Investigations
2125 Rayburn House Office Building
Washington, D.C. 20515

Dear Chairman Whitfield:

Thank you for giving the Centers for Medicare & Medicaid Services (CMS) the opportunity to testify before the Energy and Commerce Subcommittee on Oversight and Investigations regarding "A Review of Community Health Centers: Issues and Opportunities" on May 25, 2005.

Enclosed are the corrected transcript from the hearing and answers to questions submitted for the record by Congressman Dingell. A copy of this information also has been sent to his and Congressman Stupak's offices.

Your continued interest and support are essential for the Medicare program's success. If you have any questions or need additional information, please do not hesitate to contact me.

Sincerely,

Linda E. Fishman

Linda E. Fishman
Director
Office of Legislation

Enclosures

cc: The Honorable John Dingell, Ranking Member, Energy and Commerce Committee
The Honorable Bart Stupak, Ranking Member, Oversight and Investigations Subcommittee

Questions for the Record
Submitted by
Rep. John Dingell

1. In order to deal with state budget crises, many states are cutting back their Medicaid spending, and taking people off the Medicaid rolls. Missouri announced recently that it was getting out of the Medicaid program altogether. If Medicaid spending is cut, how are community health centers going to continue to provide health care for our most needy and also remain financially viable?

   Answer: In FY 2004, the total Medicaid expenditure for federally qualified health centers was $1.335 billion ($778 million Federal expenditure). The number of health centers continues to increase to currently over 1,020 centers with more than 3,876 sites. States realize that health centers provide an array of preventive and primary medical care services that beneficiaries require and have given no indication that they are considering limiting services in these settings. At the Federal level, the President's Budget does not propose any reductions in the Medicaid payment system for community health centers.

2. If, as numerous studies have found, community health centers provide better care for less money and actually cut Medicaid spending, why are we not funding even more centers? Would that not be a way to reduce Medicaid spending without cutting off beneficiaries?

   Answer: See HRSA response for this answer.

3. Dental care is one of the "optional" health services that many community health care centers provide. In Michigan, for example, it is the most frequently used service. Dental care is also the service that many states are talking about dropping. What would be the consequences for the public health if States drop dental care?

   Answer: State Medicaid agencies are committed to providing access to dental services for their eligible beneficiaries. Many states have developed innovative approaches to address the issue and among them are three examples listed below.

   MI: Michigan began contracting with Delta Dental for coverage for Medicaid children in 37 counties. These children receive the same benefits as those covered under the private Delta Dental Insurance program and the dentists are reimbursed at the same rate. In the first 12 months after this contract, there was a 32.3 % increase in the number of children receiving care in these counties over the previous year due to the expanded provider network (the existing Delta network.).

   TN: Tennessee signed a single administrative services contract with Doral Dental to be a single claims payer. and singly responsible for state-contracted deliverables. This contract to "carve out" the dental services from the state managed care contract and to increase the pay to the 75th percentile of regional dental fees resulted in a 60% increase in the provider network accepting Medicaid beneficiaries in the first 4 months.

AL: Alabama was among the first states to engage the dental provider community by forming a "Dental Task Force" to work to solve the state's declining provider enrollment. Many steps were taken to address problems cited, but among them was the decision to match the benchmark Blue Cross/ Blue Shield programs' dental fee structure in 2000. By 2002, 50,000 more children had received dental services than in 2000, and utilization was reported to be three times more than in 1998.

4. The 2004 National Healthcare Disparities Report concludes that "To reduce disparities, groups with poorer quality of care or access to care need to experience more rapid improvement in care than other groups, and this is rarely observed." Do you see any "rapid improvement" in the quality of health care or access to health care coming through your programs?

   Answer: CMS is working collaboratively with the Health Resources and Services Administration (HRSA), the Agency for Healthcare Research and Quality (AHRQ) and other public and private organizations to reduce disparities. By its very nature, the Medicaid program directly addresses health care disparities, since a disproportionate percentage of Medicaid beneficiaries are racial or ethnic minorities. Community Health Centers are an important component to reducing health care disparities because they provide access to vital health care services for medically underserved areas and medically underserved populations. Thus over the years Medicaid spending on services provided by federal qualified health centers has increased. HRSA reported that more than 63% of the populations served by CHCs in 2003 were racial/ethnic minorities.